AF841435

ENT TZ

Viva Guide in ENT Surgery

The traffic light approach

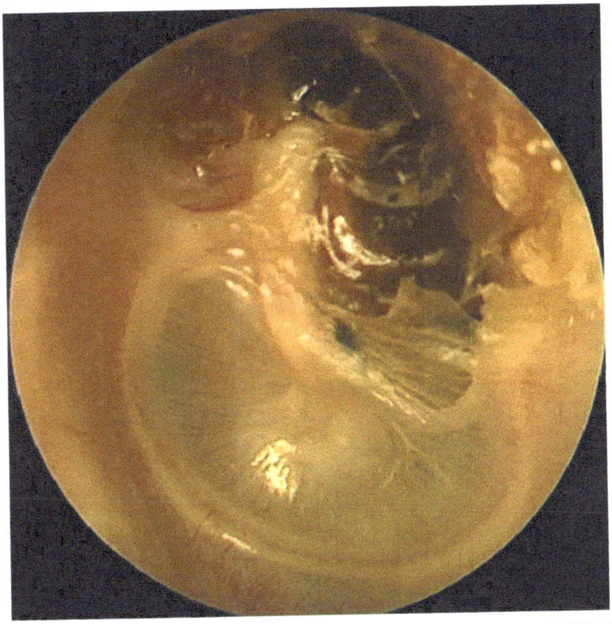

Ricardo A P Persaud | Owen Judd | Yogesh M Bhatt

Julian A Gaskin | Samuel C Leong | Paul Chatrath

Foreword by ***Professor Antony Narula*** *MA FRCS*

1st Edition 2014

FastPrint Publishing

www.fast-print.net/store.php

Viva Guide in ENT Surgery:
The traffic light approach

A catalogue record for this book is available from the British Library

ISBN 978-178456-087-4

An environmentally friendly book printed and bound in England by www.printondemand-worldwide.com

Mixed Sources
Product group from well-managed forests, and other controlled sources
www.fsc.org Cert no. TT-COC 002641
© 1996 Forest Stewardship Council

PEFC Certified
This product is from sustainably managed forests and controlled sources
www.pefc.org
PEFC/16-33-415

This book is made entirely of chain-of-custody materials

Viva Guide in ENT

The traffic light approach

RICARDO AP PERSAUD
FRCS ORL-HNS (Eng) CCT Otol. (UK)
MBBS MSB CBiol MPhil MRCS (Gen) DO-HNS
Consultant ENT Head Neck & Rhinoplastic Surgeon
Al Zahra Medical Group, Sharjah and Dubai, UAE.

OWEN JUDD
FRCS ORL-HNS (Eng) CCT Otol. (UK)
MRCP FRCS (Edin) PGDipClinEd DCH
Consultant Neurotologist and Laryngologist
Royal Derby Hospital, Derby, UK.

YOGESH M BHATT
FRCS ORL-HNS (Edin)
MB ChB (Hons) BSc (Hons) 1st Neuroscience (Lond)
Interface Fellow in Head and Neck Surgical Oncology
University Hospitals Birmingham NHS Foundation Trust, UK
Council Member for the British Association for Paediatric Otolaryngology.

JULIAN A GASKIN
FRCS ORL-HNS (Edin) CCT Otol. (UK)
MBChB DO-HNS
Fellow in Paediatric Otorhinolaryngology
University of Manchester Medical School Examiner
Royal Manchester Children's Hospital, Manchester, UK.

SAMUEL C LEONG
FRCS ORL-HNS (Edin) CCT Otol. (UK)
MPhil DOHNS MB ChB
Consultant ENT Surgeon (Rhinology & Skull Base Surgery)
University Hospital Aintree, Liverpool, UK.

PAUL CHATRATH
FRCS ORL-HNS (Eng) CCT Otol. (UK)
MB BS MA (Cantab) MD (Lond)
Consultant ENT Head Neck & Facial Plastic Surgeon
Queens University Hospital, Romford, Essex, UK
Honorary Senior Lecturer, Anglia Ruskin University, Essex, UK

Viva Guide in ENT Surgery:
The traffic light approach

CONTENTS

Preface

The *viva voce* represents the traditional test of knowledge and reasoning under fire. It continues to play a central part in Professional interviews, Diplomas and Examinations in Otorhinolaryngology worldwide, especially in Europe, North America and the Middle East.

This book has been written as a guide for those preparing for postgraduate ENT examinations. It represents the first book explicitly written to the standard of the UK FRCS specialty exit examination FRCS (ORL-HNS). It is also invaluable resource for those preparing for ENT Specialty interviews, European Board Examination or the Diploma in Otolaryngology Head Neck Surgery (DO-HNS) and MRCS (ENT) examinations.

The novel 'traffic light approach' reflects the initial introductory question at the start of the question (green), competency pass/fail question (amber) and finally the advanced question at the end (red). The mix of scenarios and/or images at the beginning of each question reflects the style of the UK postgraduate examinations. We have also incorporated a repository of the essential minute details and classification systems beloved by examiners.

Finally, as every seasoned exam goer will be aware, there is often more than one satisfactory answer to any given question and we do not intend for this guide to be used *ad verbatim*. Whilst every effort has been made to ensure that the answers given are accurate, we appreciate that clinical medicine is constantly changing and that occasionally information presented herein requires updating. We would therefore value your constructive feedback via email to ricardopersaud@enttzar.co.uk or ricardo.persaud@alzahra.com.

RAPP | OJ | YMB | JAG | SCL | PC

Aug 2014

Foreword

The *Viva Voce* continues to represent the final arbiter of sound knowledge and understanding in summative surgical assessments. This ***'Viva Guide in ENT Surgery: The traffic light approach'*** will prove to be an invaluable resource for all candidates preparing for post graduate examinations and professional ENT interviews involving clinical scenarios. It is written a format compatible with the UK Intercollegiate Fellowship Examination of the Royal College of Surgeons.

This guide book is well-illustrated and covers the breadth of the UK post-graduate curriculum in Otorhinolaryngology. The novel *'traffic light approach'* reflects the structured way examiners develop questions to test the limit of candidates understanding of important clinical topics. I have no doubt that it will succeed in being a useful tool in the armamentarium of the senior ENT Trainee as well as any clinician interested in a succinct guide of current practice, without the need of trawling through lengthy didactic textbooks. I will certainly keep a copy in my office.

Professor Antony Narula MA FRCS (Eng) FRCS (Edin)
Consultant ENT Surgeon, Imperial College Hospitals (St Mary's Hospital)
Visiting Professor, Middlesex University
Council Member Royal College of Surgeons of England
Past President of British Society of Otology
Past Board Member & Examiner Intercollegiate FRCS ORL-HNS Examination
President-Elect ENT UK (2015).

Aug 2014

"If you have no critics you will have no success"

Malcolm X

Acknowledgements

We are very grateful to Shashi Prasad, Anusha Bala and Emma Hoskison for their generous contributions and comments on the manuscripts.

CHAPTER 1

Paediatric ENT Surgery

1.1 PERIORBITAL CELLULITIS

CLINICAL PHOTOGRAPH	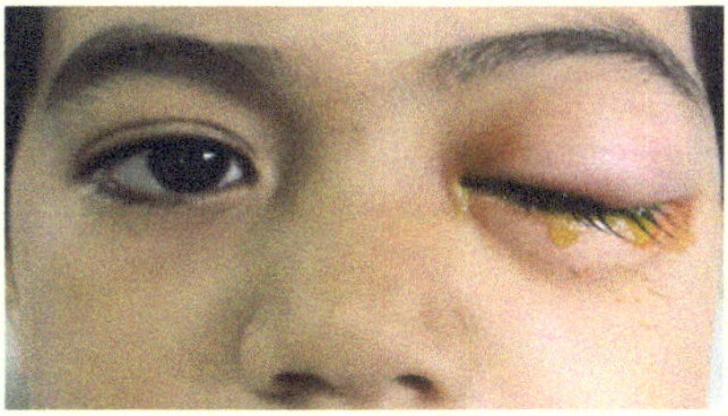

Introductory question	Answer
What is the differential diagnosis of this child in the photograph?	• Orbital cellulitis with associated sinusitis • Trauma/insect bite induced infection • Dysthyroid eye disease • Orbital pseudo-tumour • Mucocele • Non-accidental injury

Competency question(s)	Answer
How would you manage this patient?	• This is a sight threatening emergency and is best managed together with an ophthalmologist and depends upon the grade of the infection. • **History** – determine likelihood of orbital cellulitis and associated sinusitis. Pain, diplopia, impaired vision, duration of symptoms. DH/allergy. • **Examination** – determine likelihood of post-septal disease by identifying proptosis, diplopia, chemosis or pain on eye movement. Assess visual acuity with Snellen chart and red desaturation with Ishihara plates. Gross test of CN2 function using swinging light test for RAPD. Bilateral eye signs raise possibility of cavernous sinus thrombosis • **Investigations –** CT imaging of nose and paranasal sinuses, orbits and brain with contrast if: 1. Suspecting post-septal disease (Chandler's II to V) 2. No response to 24 hours of IV antibiotics 3. Visual acuity cannot be assessed adequately or routinely • MR brain with contrast if intracranial complication suspected. • **Treatment** – IV antibiotic guided by

	local protocol and intranasal steroid and decongestants. Initially, hourly eye observations and 4-hourly neuro-obs until evidence of disease resolution. • Thin medial subperiosteal collections may be managed conservatively if regular reliable acuity assessment is available. All other collections must be drained immediately. • ***Drainage*** may be performed externally to allow drain insertion or if expertise available, endonasally. • Maxillary antrum may be washed out and aspirate sent for MC&S
Advanced question(s)	**Answer**
What if there is a forehead swelling in this child?	• This is likely to represent a subperiosteal collection of an osteomyelitic anterior table of the frontal sinus or Potts Puffy Tumour. • This condition is associated with intracranial complications in 33% of cases and demands an MR brain with contrast enhancement and repeat assessment as symptoms dictate. • IV antibiotic treatment should have good bone penetrance and duration suitable for treating an osteomyelitic process. • Surgical goals are to drain the pus – direct incision may lead to fistulation

	and frontal sinus surgery may be hazardous. Frontal sinus trephine may represent an effective compromise. Bony sequestra occasionally require open debridement.

1.2 HYPOVOLAEMIC SHOCK

SCENARIO **(no clinical photograph)**	You are asked to see a 3 yr old boy who underwent adeno-tonsillectomy for OSA 2 hours previously. He is pale and aggitated but apyrexial with a heart rate of 165bpm, respiratory rate 40/min and capillary refill (CR) time of 5 seconds.

Introductory question	**Answer**
What is your clinical diagnosis?	• Hypovolaemic shock (uncompensated)
Competency question(s)	**Answer**
What is shock and how would you manage this child?	• Shock refers to systemic organ dysfunction resulting from hypo-perfusion and/or hypo-oxygenation. In this case it is from hypovolaemia due to blood loss (cf. dehydration) • When compensated blood flow to vital organs is preserved but the child may be agitated with raised HR and CR. Low BP is a pre-terminal sign of decompensation and circulatory collapse may quickly follow.

	• Seek input from an experienced anaesthetist/paediatrician and simultaneously assess and treat the child using APLS protocol in an appropriate setting eg RESUS bay, theatre recovery or HDU with oxygen and fluids. • A – clear clots and administer high flow oxygen, B – assess effort, efficacy and effect of breathing, C – reassess signs and urine output and obtain 2 wide bore IV access lines whilst obtaining blood for cross-match, FBC, coagulopathy screen. • Administer a 20ml/kg normal saline (0.9%) bolus and check for response. If bleeding continues and once 40ml/kg had been administered, colloid/blood products must be given next. • Once stabilised the child should be taken to theatre to formally control the bleed.
Advanced question(s)	**Answer**
How would your management be changed if the child was pyrexial? How would it be changed if IV access could not be obtained?	• Pyrexia might suggest an infective component i.e. septic shock. If the child was not penicillin allergic, I would administer cefotaxime at 80mg/kg. • If no IV access was achievable immediately, obtain intra-osseous access. With a knee flexed at 30degree over a towel clean the skin over either antero-medial surface of tibia 3cm below the tibial tuberosity or antero-lateral femur 3cm above the lateral condyle.

	Rotate an 18G IO needle at 90 degrees to the bone until a 'give' is felt. Aspirated to confirm position and 20ml of crystalloid pushed through the syringe and line secured.

1.3 EPIGLOTITIS

SCENARIO **(no clinical photograph)**	You are asked to see a 3 yr old with a 12 hours history of sore throat and noisy breathing. On examination she is pyrexial and drooling.

Introductory question	Answer
What is your differential diagnosis?	• Epiglottitis • Laryngo-tracheo-bronchitis (croup) • Deep neck space abscess • Airway foreign body • Severe pharyngo-tonsillitis (bacterial or viral aetiology)
Competency question(s)	**Answer**
How would you manage this patient?	• **History** – Taken whilst making primary ABC assessment in line with APLS principles. Establish rapidity of symptom onset or any history of choking. Vaccination history. Social history ie children at home. DH/allergies esp. antibiotics. • **Examination** – Without further upsetting

	child by oral examination or cannulation, assess effort and efficacy of breathing including phase of stridor, use of accessory muscles, tracheal tug, grunting. Desaturation is a pre-terminal event. Ask family to hold nebulised adrenaline in oxygen close to child. Further assessments should be made in theatre. • **Investigations** – With the assistance of a senior anaesthetist the child should be taken to theatre with age appropriate and smaller oro and naso-tracheal tubes, ventilating bronchoscope and paediatric pharyngoscope/Hopkins rod endoscope and tracheostomy tray. Intubation with spontaneously ventilating inhalational anaesthetic. • **Treatment** – IV ceftriaxone administered and child to remain intubated on paediatric ITU until tube leak present or reassessed with laryngoscope in 48hours. Sepsis treated in conjunction with paediatric intensivists.
Advanced question(s)	**Answer**
What is Heliox?	• It is a gaseous mixture of helium and oxygen typically 79 percent and 21 percent, respectively. It is less dense than either oxygen or room air and has properties of low resistance laminar airflow, despite the increased flow velocity which occurs as a consequence

	of airway narrowing.
What is its role in upper airway obstruction?	• It represents a temporising measure which facilitates ventilation and may reduce the likelihood of exhaustion before the airway is secured by intubation, tracheostomy or other therapies. Its function is to minimise the risk of hypercapnia and CO_2 narcosis/acidosis.

1.4 FOREIGN BODY WHEEZING

SCENARIO **(followed by a radiological image)**	A&E referral: You are called by the paediatricians to see a 2 year old boy with a 6 month history of intermittent wheezing, occasional cough and sneezing. His parents became concerned after he developed a high temperature over the weekend.

Introductory question	Answer
What is your differential diagnosis and how would you assess the child?	• **Differential diagnosis**: FB inhalation, asthma exacerbation, severe allergy, croup, bronchiolitis, undiagnosed subglottic stenosis • **Assessment**: Start with ABC. Then ***History***: FB ingestion, history of URTI prior to onset, asthma, eczema, food allergies, previous history of pyrexia-induced convulsions. Any voice disturbance. Problems at birth – premature, SCBU, intubation and duration. ***Examination***: Recessions, listen to chest (is it wheezing from LRT, a stertorous noise or stridor); examine nose, FNE may be difficult in this age group ***Investigations***: CXR and FBC and differential, based on the history

Competency question(s)	Answer
Here is the CXR. Describe what you see 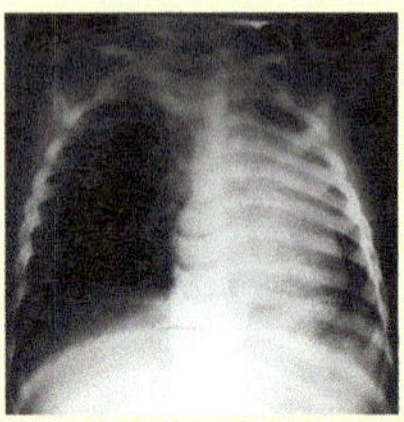	CXR shows evidence of hyperinflation of the right lung with mediastinal shift to the left. This is most likely to be due to a foreign body in the right main bronchus having a ball valve effect
How would you remove it?	With optical forceps and a ventilating bronchoscope. The use of 1:10,000 adrenaline injected through the suction port is very helpful to aid visualisation (by vasoconstricting the blood vessels).
Advanced question(s)	**Answer**
What would you do if you cannot remove it?	• Enlist help of respiratory colleagues for bronchoscopy, failing that, option of last resort is to consult with thoracic team for possible thoracotomy, usually reserved for patients with serious/life threatening complications such as airway obstruction or empyema.

1.5 ACUTE OTITIS MEDIA (AOM)

CLINICAL PHOTOGRAPH	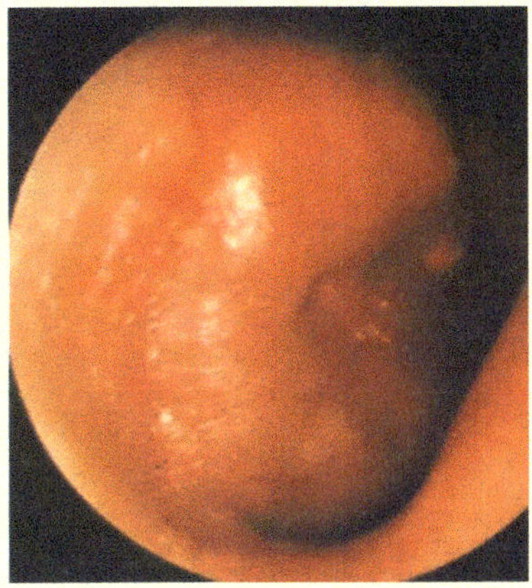

Introductory question	Answer
A 5yr old presents with a 3 day history of otalgia and pyrexia. You examine the ear which looks like the clinical photograph above. Please describe what you see?	• An otoscopic photograph of a right tympanic membrane with evidence of bulging and erythema consistent with acute otitis media.

Competency question(s)	Answer
How would you manage this child?	• Management guided by an acknowledgement that AOM is typically self-limiting simply requiring supportive treatment. Treatment chosen in partnership with parent. History and examination used to determine the appropriateness of supportive therapy vs delayed antibiotics vs immediate antibiotics.(SIGN Guidelines for AOM, 2003) • Supportive treatment may be considered in those over 2 yr old and an explanation of likely duration of symptoms should be given (4days) and an option given to take antibiotic therapy if symptoms persisting beyond 2-3days or symptoms worsening. • Children with or at risk of complications should be given immediate antibiotic therapy. These include severely ill children, those with a history of complications, the immunodeficient, craniofacial dysmorphism predisposing to Eustachian tube dysfunction (Down syndrome or cleft palate), children under 2 yrs with bilateral AOM and those with a cochlear implant. • First line antibiotic may be 5 days of amoxicillin. Second line therapy is co-amoxiclav if child not responding to 3 days of first line treatment or recently treatment with antibiotics, high local

	prevalence of beta-lactamase producing organisms or at higher risk of complications. Ensure Prevenar (Pneumococcal Conjugate Vaccine) has been considered.
Advanced question(s)	**Answer**
What is the role of myringotomy in the treatment of AOM?	• No randomised studies have demonstrated the benefit of tympanocentesis in the routine treatment of AOM. • A firm indication may be children with a complication of AOM or impending complication. A relative indication may be the severely ill child not responding to antibiotic therapy. • Tympanocentesis may be performed under GA or LA using a 23g needle mounted on a 2cm3 syringe. • Elective myringotomy and tympanostomy tube insertion has been shown to reduce the rate of AOM in children with recurrent AOM.

1.6 ACUTE MASTOIDITIS

CLINICAL PHOTOGRAPH	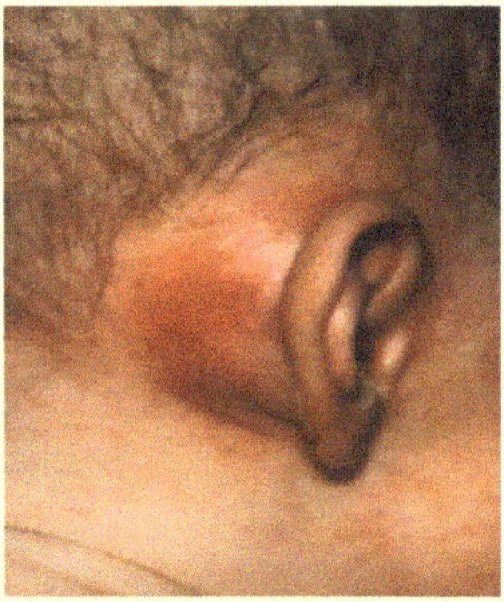

Introductory question	Answer
What are the differential diagnoses?	This is a clinical photograph showing a right post auricular swelling with pinna proptosis. The differential diagnoses are: • Subperiosteal collection complicating acute mastoiditis • Post-auricular lymphadenopathy • Post-auricular soft-tissue infection • Pinna/mastoid trauma

Competency question(s)	Answer
How would you investigate and manage this patient?	• **History** – duration of otalgia, otorrhoea, type and duration of antibiotic therapy. History of AOM complications. DH/allergies. • **Examination** – assess for signs of mastoiditis including dull TM, posterior canal wall sag, and tenderness of antrum on palpating the cymba concha. Fluctuant post-aural collection. Assess for intra- and extra-temporal complications including AVPU, meningism and facial nerve function. • **Investigations –** CT imaging with contrast of the temporal bone and brain to help exclude co-existing intra-cranial complications. • **Treatment** – Trial of IV ceftriaxone if child not grossly unwell or if no collection. If otherwise or not responding to 24hrs trial of therapy then incision and drainage and cortical mastoidectomy with drain and myringotomy +/- grommet insertion. Care not to extend post-aural incision below level of floor of ear canal due to risk of superficial facial nerve. Send pus for MC+S.

Advanced question(s)	Answer
Despite the above treatment the child continues to experience picket fence spikes of pyrexia. A CT scan is performed. Please describe its findings and explain how would you manage this? 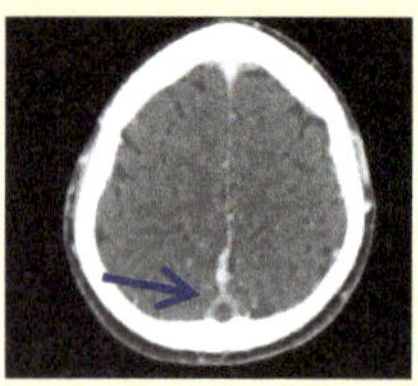 **Figure 1.6a**. Delta sign	• The scan in figure 1.6a demonstrates the enhancement of the wall of the sagittal sinus with a contrast void in its lumen. This is the 'delta sign' and suggests a cerebral venous sinus thrombosis. • Liaise with a microbiologist, to ensure adequacy of antibiotic therapy with intra-cranial penetrance, and a senior otologist. • This thrombosis may result in raised ICP causing 'otitic hydrocephalus'. The child should be managed with a paediatrician and nursed with neurological observation. Anti-coagulation may be indicated in the presence of an extending or symptomatic thrombosis. The presence of local cerebritis may increase the risk of anticoagulation induced haemorrhage.

1.7 NEONATAL NASAL OBSTRUCTION

SCENARIO **(no clinical photograph)**	Whilst in the outpatient clinic you received a call for the Obstetrician who just delivered a baby. The newborn appears blue but becomes pinks on crying. The Obstetrician is concerned that the baby may have an airway problem and would like you to come urgently.

Introductory question	Answer
What is your differential diagnosis?	• Bilateral choanal atresia, • Nasal mass (glioma, encephalocele, meningoencephalocele, nasolacrimal duct tumours etc) • Piriform aperture stenosis • Severe neonatal rhinitis
Competency question(s)	**Answer**
How would you manage the case?	• **History** –brief neonatal history whilst inserting and securing a oropharyngeal airway and orogastric tube for feeding. • **Examination** – try to pass a fine bore catheter through the nose, listen for

	sounds on stethoscope held under nose. Check for misting on a cold Lack spatula placed under the nose. • **Investigations –** Axial CT scan through the post nasal space after decongesting and suctioning of nose to confirm diagnosis. • **If bilateral choanal atresia is present I would think of** CHARGE Syndrome and request an ECHO to rule out cardiac abnormalities, Ultrasound scan of kidneys to rule out renal problems. Later, slit lamp examination of eyes (coloboma) as well as OAEs and ABR • **Treatment** – surgery ASAP to create and maintain patent posterior choanae. Can be done endonasally under direct vision by using a 120 degrees rigid Hopkins rod in the mouth. The alternative is the trans-palatine approach, which involves removal the posterior part of the vomer. A soft tube splint for up to 6 weeks is necessary.
Advanced question(s)	**Answer**
What is CHARGE?	• CHARGE is an acronym for **C**oloboma, **H**eart abnormality, **A**tresia of choana, **R**etardation of growth, **G**enital/urinary abnormality and **E**ar abnormality.
Is CHARGE an association, a	• CHARGE is a syndrome, rather than an association, because the cause has been identified (mutations of CHD7 gene on

syndrome or a sequence?	chromosome 8). • An association is when the cause is unknown whilst a sequence is when one abnormality leads to another eg Pierre Robin sequence.

1.8 RETROPHARYNGEAL ABSCESS

SCENARIO	You are asked to see a 3yrs-old child with a 24 hour history of worsening snoring, temperature and reduced oral intake. She exhibits a reduced range of neck movement.

Introductory question	Answer
What is your differential diagnosis?	• Retropharyngeal collection • Prevertebral collection • Parapharyngeal collection • Neck trauma
Competency question(s)	**Answer**
The A+E department requested a lateral cervical spine plain x-ray in extension. What is the likely pathophysiology for this condition and how would you manage this	• The film demonstrates AP thickness of the pre-vertebral space in excess of a vertebral body width with loss of cervical lordosis (normal prevertebral thickness C1-C4 = 7mm, C4-C8 = 17mm). Suggests retro-pharyngeal or pre-vertebral space collection. Often secondary to suppurative lymphadenopathy of the retropharyngeal Rouviere node in children under 4yrs of age.

patient? 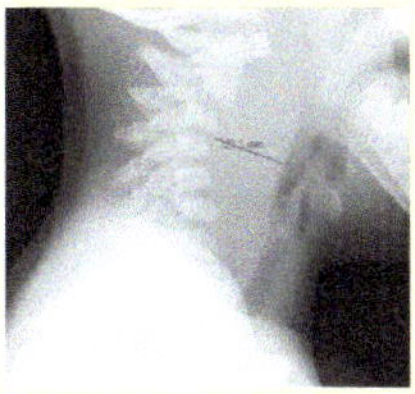	• **History** – Blunt trauma, foreign body ingestion, URTI, tuberculosis contact, DH/allergy. • **Examination** – Effort and efficacy of breathing noting stertor/stridor and administration of high flow humidified oxygen by parent. Careful oral assessment for parapharyngeal & retropharyngeal swelling. Associated neurology or chest signs. • **Investigation –** cross-sectional imaging if symptoms do not settle within 24 hours of IV antibiotics or evidence of frank collection. Allows planning of route of drainage and identification of complications. • **Treatment –** analgesia and IV antibiotics. Manage sepsis with paediatrician. Drainage if signs of airway compromise or no response to antibiotics. Liaise with senior anaesthetist for naso-tracheal intubation following gaseous induction taking care not to rupture collection. Oro-tracheal intubation over a rigid endoscope may be required. Trans-oral drainage is ideal first line route. Monitor for signs of recurrence of complications.
Advanced question(s)	**Answer**
What are the principles of draining a retro-pharyngeal	• An extensive collection is best drained externally in order to allow insertion of a drain, obtain tissue for histology and thoroughly irrigate the cavity. Trans-

collection extending into the thorax?	cervical incision at hyoid level retracting SCM laterally and rotating larynx and pharynx medially following ligation of middle thyroid vein. • Collections above T4 will drain through a trans-cervical incision. Those below will require discussion with a paediatric surgeon regarding need for trans-thoracic drainage. • Repeat imaging is essential to ensure resolution and management with a paediatrician in a level 2 or 3 environment.

1.9 JUVENILE RESPIRATORY PAPILLOMATOSIS

SCENARIO	You are referred a 4 year old boy in whom the parents are concerned about persistent hoarseness.

Introductory question	Answer
What is your differential diagnosis?	1. Vocal cord nodules 2. Respiratory papilloma 3. Extra-oesophageal reflux 4. Vocal cord palsy 5. Chronic laryngitis
Competency question(s)	**Answer**
What is recurrent respiratory papillomatosis? How would you manage this child?	• An acquired condition of viral aetiology chiefly HPV 6 and HPV 11 serotypes and typified by the presence of papillomata within the laryngo-tracheal tract and beyond. Juvenile onset RRP tends to be more aggressive than adult onset disease, but may spontaneously resolve in adolescence. The presence of papillomas beyond the vocal folds suggests metaplasia of the respiratory

	epithelium to squamous epithelium. • The primary goal is making the diagnosis with flexible and ultimately rigid airway endoscopy to stage the disease. Given that there is no cure for the condition the management goal is to reduce morbidity by reducing papilloma bulk to optimise voice and airway whilst minimising collateral damage to normal structures. • Close cooperation with the anaesthetist to manage the shared airway with techniques including: spontaneous ventilation, intermittent apnoea and jet ventilation techniques. • Debulking techniques include: Cold steel, CO_2 laser ablation (risk stenosis or webbing with overuse as well as spread of virus to surgeon from the laser smoke) and microdebrider (the preferred method of most units). • Adjuvant therapy may include alpha-interferon for aggressive disease. Cidofovir, a cytosine nucleoside analogue, has been topically intra-operatively but concerns have been raised about carcinogenic potential. • Tracheostomy is sometimes employed in children whose disease presents a risk of airway loss, but should be regarded as a last resort as a tracheostomy has precipitate distal airway involvement of papillomata.

Advanced question(s)	Answer
Describe the role of HPV vaccination in the management of RRP	• National HPV vaccination strategies have been established in the UK. The first vaccine Cervarix was designed to vaccinate against cervical cancer causing serotypes 16 and 18. • The present vaccine Gardasil is quadrivalent covering the additional RRP serotypes 6, 11. It is offered to all girls aged 12-13yrs and administered as 0.5ml intramuscularly at a 0, 2 and 6 month schedule. All three must be given within 12months with the second at least 1 month after the first and the third at least 3 months after the second. • It is not licenced for the treatment for active HPV disease i.e. pre-existing RRP. • With the apparent rise in HPV-related oropharyngeal cancer, the vaccine may be given to boys in the future.

1.10 PRE-AURICULAR SINUS

CLINICAL PHOTOGRAPH	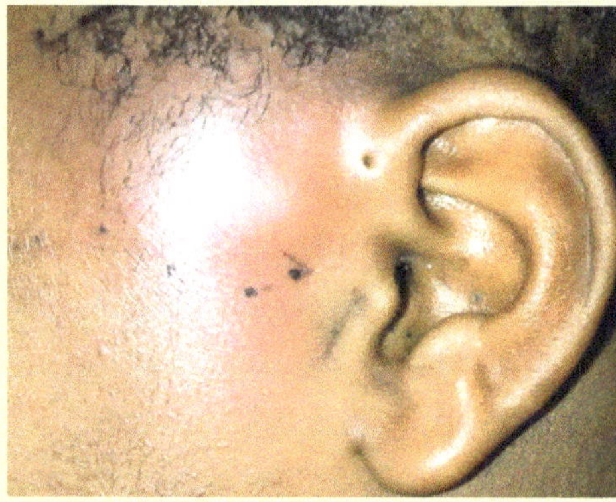

Introductory question	Answer
What is the diagnosis?	• Infected pre-auricular sinus
Competency question(s)	**Answer**
Describe the embryology of this anomaly and how you manage this. Describe the surgical	• Pre-auricular sinus arises from failure of fusion of the Hillocks of His from the first branchial arch with attachment to the cartilage of the root of helix. 25-50% are bilateral and associated with Syndromes e.g. Branchio-oto-renal (BOR) syndrome. • Acute infections treated with directed

techniques used to electively treat this condition	antibiotics or I+D if abscess. • Elective assessment of EAC for connecting pits suggesting first branchial arch anomaly. Inspect contralateral ear and neck for second arch cyst/sinus. • Consider renal tract us/s for BOR syndrome if pre-auricular sinus and one of the following: 1. FH of hearing loss, renal anomaly or BOR syndrome 2. A second dysmorphic feature 3. Maternal gestational diabetes • Non-infected pits typically remain un-infected and do not require further assessment or surgery. • The 3 techniques include: 1. Simple sinusectomy 2. Wide local excision by a supra-auricular approach 3. 'Inside-out' technique • **Sinusectomy** involves elliptical skin incision around the punctum and excision of tract using probe +/- methylene blue. 20-40% risk of recurrence • **Wide local excision** (Emery) includes an elliptical incision extended in a curvilear fashion above the pinna. An *en-bloc* specimen is removed with a cuff of perichondrium from helical root and tissue removed to the depth of the

	temporalis fascia remaining posterior to the temporal artery to minimise injury to the facial nerve branches. 5% risk of recurrence. • **The inside-out technique** (Jensma) combines the wide-local incision approach and surgical magnification with opening of the tract to follow each branch of the sinus.
Advanced question(s)	**Answer**
What is the embryology of a preauricular sinus?	• First arch not a first cleft abnormality. • The ear is formed by 6 hillocks of His derived from the first and second **arches** • Failure of complete closure of the hillocks of His results in sinus formation

1.11 MICROTIA

CLINICAL PHOTOGRAPH	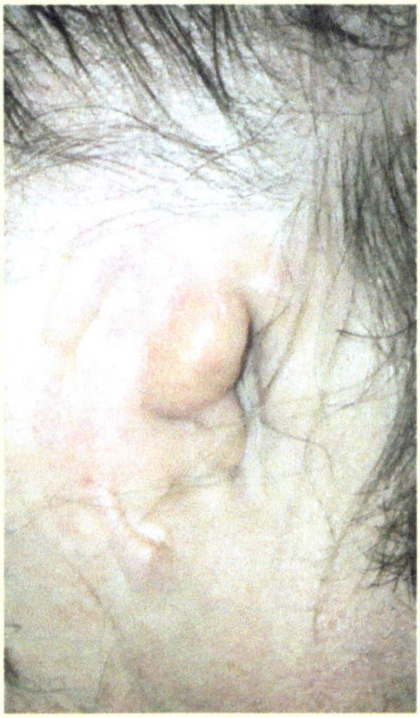

Introductory question	Answer
What is the name of this condition?	Microtia (grade 3)
Competency question(s)	**Answer**
What are the issues related to this condition and	**Functional issues** –hearing loss usually CHL up to 60dB due to canal atresia +/- ossicular

how would you manage them?	dysfunction. It is important to determine the status of the other ear and the presence of other abnormalities, for example is the patient syndromic (Golderhar, CHARGE). For rehabilitation of hearing loss, consider a trial of bone conduction hearing aid on soft band and later BAHA **Cosmetic issues** –surgical reconstruction or prosthesis. Only a few centres achieve good results with surgery, which involves multiple staged procedures. Bone anchored prosthesis is probably the preferred option.
Advanced question(s)	**Answer**
What factors should be considered if surgical reconstruction is required?	Timing of surgery is crucial. Ideally the patient should be fully involved in the decision making. In the case of a child around age 6-7 when the rib is matured enough to harvest cartilage. The size of the normal pinna may be used as a 'template' Imaging of the ossicles and facial nerve to determine possible abnormal anatomy which may make surgery very challenging. Multidiscipilinary team involvement

1.12 OTITIS MEDIA WITH EFFUSION (GLUE EAR)

SCENARIO **(no clinical photograph)**	GP referral Please could you see this 4 year old girl whose parents have concerns about her hearing.

Introductory question	Answer
How would you initially assess this child?	**History**: Length of history (>3months), speech delay, balance disturbance, pain, history of AOM, nasal problems/nasal block, snoring/OSA, sore throats, chest infections, birth history, other infections / immune deficits. **Examination**: otoscopy, nasal airflow, oral cavity. **Investigations**: PTA and tymps since she is 4 years old.
Competency question(s)	**Answer**
This is what the ear looks like (on both sides). Tell me what you see.	This is a clinical photograph of the left tympanic membrane showing otitis media with effusion because of the retracted tympanic membrane, cloudy appearance and neoannulus; the hyperaemia of the tympanic

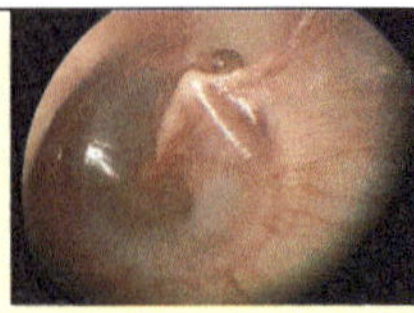 What are the non-surgical options for treating glue ear?	membrane probably indicates a recent URTI. Watch and wait (at least 3months). Medications: No evidence that decongestants, antibiotics or antihistamines are beneficial. Steroids may be helpful but has significant side effects. Autoinflation such as with the Otovent balloon has been shown to improve effusions over a 2 week to 3 month period but evidence for longer term benefit is lacking. Bearing in mind the complications associated with ventilation tube insertion, many clinicians consider autoinflation techniques particularly useful in cases of unilateral middle ear effusions. Hearing aids should also be considered. Adherence to the 2008 NICE guidelines are often required.
Advanced question(s)	**Answer**
How would you manage a patient who has had 3 sets of conventional grommets in the past, and a t-tube which has fallen out, who develops a further middle ear effusion?	Reassess with particular attention to nasal function and pathology, also the patient's immune status should be considered. Examine the ears carefully for the presence of retraction pockets. **Options**: optimise nasal function, medical (hearing aid), surgical – another t-tube, extra-annular t-tube.

1.13 BRANCHIAL CLEFT SINUS

SCENARIO **(no clinical photograph)**	You are referred a 6year-old boy with a discharging sinus on the lateral aspect of the neck behind the angle of the mandible.

Introductory question	Answer
What is your differential diagnosis?	Branchial cleft sinus Lateral thyroglossal duct anomaly Mycobacterial disease Actinomycosis
Competency question(s)	**Answer**
How would you manage this patient?	**History –** Pre-existing punctum or cyst. Prior local surgery. FH of Branchio-Oto-Renal syndrome. **Examination –** inspect EAC for communication and contra-lateral neck for sinus/cyst. **Investigation –** fistulogram of tract. MRI considered. Barium swallow if type 3 or 4 cleft anamoly is suspected. **Treatment –** definitive treatment is excision

	during quiescence. Type 1 sinus is EAC duplication and approached through parotidectomy incision with facial nerve monitoring. Type 2 sinus traced between internal/external carotid above CN12 into tonsil in older children via step-ladder incision.
Advanced question(s)	**Answer**
Describe the presentation of type 3 and 4 cleft sinus and its operative management	Type 3 and 4 sinuses both communicate with the pyriform fossa and often the ipsilateral thyroid gland and may present with recurrent suppurative thyroiditis. Type 3 sinus extends between CN10 and common carotid piercing the thyro-hyoid membrane. Type 4 sinuses are very uncommon and run a course parallel to the recurrent laryngeal nerve by pierce the cricothyroid membrane. Surgical options include excision of tract +/- hemi-thyroidectomy or endoscopic cautery of the sinus opening into piriform fossa in young children.

1.14 DROOLING

SCENARIO **(and clinical photo)**	You are asked to see a 4 yrs-old child. His mother is concerned about his face and clothes being regularly soiled by saliva 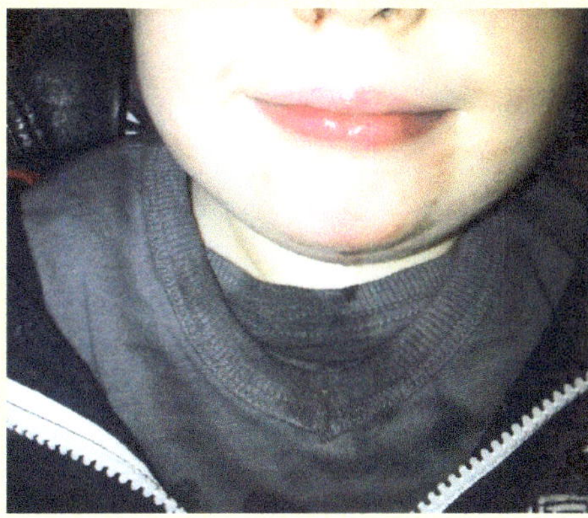

Introductory question	Answer
What is the clinical name for this condition and at what age is this condition considered abnormal?	Drooling/sialorrhoea Drooling may be physiological up to 5 years old. Due to overflow, not over-production. Associated with poorer oromotor coordination in younger children.

Competency question(s)	Answer
How would you examine him specifically?	History and examination: number of bibs, clothing changes per day. Oromotor coordination/ control Physical and mental development: ?age appropriate. Dental problems (?has the dentist been involved) Impact on family and quality of life.
Which groups of patients have drooling?	Chronic drooling: Cerebral palsy, syndromic (e.g. Trisomy-21), children on anti-convulsants. Acute drooling: foreign body, infections e.g. epiglotitis, tonsilitis, gingivitis.
How would you manage this child?	Management should be guided by the cause and severity of drooling and an appreciation of the psychosocial impact. Management of a drooling child is challenging and requires a multi-disciplinary approach. Involve the community paediatrician, paediatric neurologist, dentist, physiotherapist etc. Severity may be graded by the presence of peri-oral skin maceration and the number of clothes changes per day for the soiling. **Investigation** includes MDT assessment of head control, dental malocclusion and swallowing dysfunction. Assess for causes of hypersecretion eg dental carries and causes of incomplete lip seal eg macroglossia.

	Conservative: sitting positions, changing food texture, oromotor exercises, cognitive behavioural therapy Medical: Hyoscine, glycopyrolate Botulinum toxin injection. This is normally available at tertiary paediatric units. Can be injected under ultrasound guidance and can be repeated. Effect wears off after 3 - 4 months. Surgery: tonsillectomy, salivary gland surgery.
Advanced question(s)	**Answer**
How would this child's co-morbidity affect your surgical options?	Surgical options include submandibular duct re-positioning, submandibular +/- sublingual gland excision and parotid duct ligation. Duct re-routing has low morbidity but may increase the tendency for salivary aspiration if pre-existing dysphagia. Associated risks of re-routing include ranula formation. Bilateral SMG removal may increase likelihood of dental caries because of reduced protective effect of saliva. Parotid duct tie off carries risk of sialocele formation. Aspiration needs to be excluded before embarking on surgery.

1.15 LARYNGOMALACIA

SCENARIO **(no clinical photograph)**	You are asked to see a 10-week-old boy who mother is concerned with persistent noisy breathing.

Introductory question	Answer
What is your differential diagnosis for noisy breathing?	**Stertor** may be due nasal obstruction caused by piriform aperture stenosis, choanal atresia, nasal and post-nasal mass, Pharyngeal obstruction due to large tonsils, poor muscle tone, glossoptosis +/- mandibular hypoplasia **Stridor** may be due to supraglottic pathology, including laryngomalacia, cysts or papillomata, Glottic pathology including vocal cord palsy, glottis web, cysts, papillomata, Subglottic pathology including stenosis, cysts, haemangioma, Tracheal including vascular ring/sling, congenital anomalies, tracheobronchomalacia.
Competency question(s)	**Answer**
What is the most likely diagnosis and how would you manage this	Laryngomalacia is the most common cause of chronic stridor in infancy. **History –** Age at onset, rate of progression,

patient? When would you perform direct laryngoscopy?	impact on feeding, choking, apnoea, and cyanosis. Birth history as well as number and duration intubations. Neuromuscular disorders. **Examination** – effort and efficacy of ventilation including nasal flare, tracheal tug, chest recession. Phase and type of noise: pharyngeal stertor improved with jaw thrust or laryngotracheal stridor. Nasal cold spatula testing. Oral examination – cleft palate and glossoptosis. Neck – mass. Top to toe exam for cutaneous haemangioma. Growth chart from 'red book'. A child with a history consistent with simple laryngomalacia with inspiratory stridor, thriving without prior tracheal intubation or haemangioma may be managed with regular outpatient review, an outpatient supraglottic examination and treatment of co-existing extra-oesophageal reflux. **Direct laryngoscopy** should be performed if history of intubation, haemangioma, diagnostic uncertainty, biphasic stridor or failure to thrive.
Advanced question(s)	**Answer**
The child undergoes rigid laryngo-tracheo-bronchoscopy. A mid-tracheal compression is	Secondary airway lesions are present in over 50% of children with severe laryngomalacia who require aryepiglottoplasty. I would assess for any dynamic component of the narrowing including deterioration on expiration i.e. tracheomalacia, pulsatility or

noted. What is the significance of this and how would you manage this child?	fixed narrowing which may result from a complete tracheal ring. Any possibility of extrinsic compression should be investigated with CT thorax which in young infants may be performed by 'feed and wrap' techniques or in older children may require sedation using local protocol eg oral chloral hydrate +/- rectal paraldehyde. Rarely infants may decompensate with sedatives and may need imaging under general anaesthetic with intubation. Vascular compression due to complete rings include double aortic arch causing posterolateral compression of the distal trachea, right aortic arch with left ligamentum arteriosum. Incomplete rings may be caused by aberrant innominate artery compression of the anterior wall of the upper trachea. Compression may also be caused by anomalous left or right pulmonary artery (pulmonary artery sling).

1.16 DOWN SYNDROME

SCENARIO (clinical photograph)	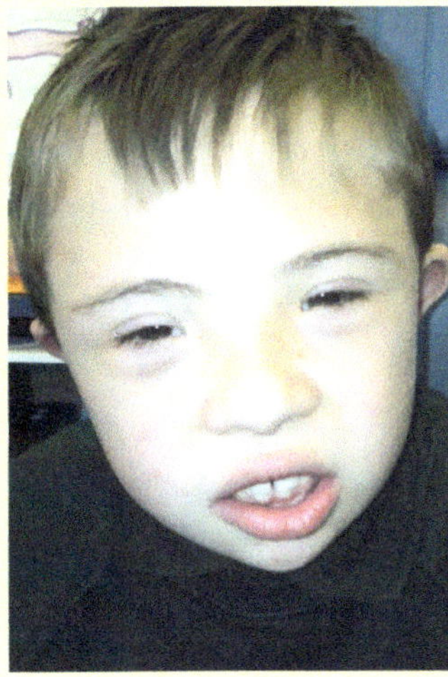

Introductory question	Answer
This young boy just moved into the area. What syndrome is he affected by?	• This young boy has classical features of Down syndrome; these include upslanting palpebral fissures with epicanthic folds, small low set ears, wide nasal bridge and open mouth because of macroglossia.
Competency question(s)	**Answer**
Why might he	• Patients with Down syndrome may have

come to see you as an ENT surgeon?	disorders pertaining to the Ear, Nose, Throat and Neck. • **Ears:** Small low set pinnae, Ear canal stenosis, ***Conductive hearing loss,*** Wax impaction**,** Otitis Media with Effusion (OME) (decreased immunity, hypotonic palate, Eustachian tube dysfunction)**,** Cholesteatoma**,** Ossicular abnormalities (deformed stapes, thickened malleus)**,** Up to 80% facial nerve dehiscence (wide angle 2nd genu)**,** Sensorineural hearing loss in 21% of patients under 20 years of age, 55% of patients over 20 years (labyrinthine hypoplasia, small bony island LSCC) • **Nose:** Structure (cosmesis) and function, Flat, Nasal congestion (increased URTI), drooling, Small narrow nasopharynx (OME), Sinus hypoplasia (increased sinonasal disease), hypotonicity of pharynx • **Throat (inc Airway):** macroglossia, Obstructive Sleep Apnoea, no lip seal, drooling**,** subglottic narrowing**,** recurrent croup (reduced immunity/immature T and B cell function)**,** smaller endotracheal tube needed • **Neck:** Atlantoaxial instability (10%); this is relevant to Tonsillectomy**,** Ear Surgery. Pre-op x-ray neck +/- neurology opinion may be needed. Patients should be operated in the neutral position.

Advanced question(s)	Answer
Why is there an increased incidence of CROUP in children with Down syndrome?	• May be related to subglottic narrowing (Steeple's sign on X-ray) and/or dysfunctional immune system with reduced/immature T and B cell function.

1.17 HAEMANGIOMAS

SCENARIO **(no clinical photograph)**	You are asked to see a 2 month old infant with noisy breathing worse when crying and associated with feeding difficulty. There is a quiet biphasic stridor at rest. You notice a red lesion on his chin.

Introductory question	Answer
What is your differential diagnosis?	• The nature of stridor suggests subglottic pathology. • The association with a red facial lesion suggest a haemangioma or a vascular malformation. • The differential includes subglottic stenosis (primary or acquired), subglottic web/cyst and foreign body
Competency question(s)	**Answer**
Assuming you suspect a subglottic haemangioma how would you manage this	• **History** – exclude associated diagnosis eg choking episodes and previous intubations. Birth and developmental history. Assess impact on feeding. • **Examination** – Note any dysmorphism and degree of respiratory effort i.e.

patient? What are the side-effects of propanolol?	tug/recession and efficacy i.e. oxygen saturation. Assess nasal patency, oral examination and fibre optic supraglottic assessment in clinic if available. Top to toe exam for haemangioma of infancy. Growth chart for failure to thrive. • **Investigations –** Will require rigid airway examination under GA for diagnosis whilst spontaneous ventilating with inhalational anaesthesia via nasopharyngeal airway. • **Treatment** – the pathology may grow over the first few months of life. Most patients with haemangioma do not require treatment but functionally impairing lesions (especially subglottic) may be treated with propranolol, systemic or intra-lesional steroids. Open/laser resection, tracheostomy and historically intra-lesional vincristine. • Propranolol is a non-selective beta-antagonist, therefore bradycardia and potential heart failure, hypoglycaemia, bronchospasm and hypotension are possible side effects.
Advanced question(s)	**Answer**
What are the proposed mechanisms of action of propanolol.	1. Vasoconstriction leads to colour change and softening of the haemangioma 2. Down regulation of RAF-mitogen-activated protein kinase pathway 3. Decreased expression of VEGF and b-FGF

What dose of propranolol would you prescribe?	genes 4. Induction of apoptosis of capillary endothelial cells. • Start with 0.16mg/kg/day to max 2mg/kg/day; initial treatment should be in hospital as cardiac monitoring is required as well as paediatrician input for possible hypoglycaemia • Note that 10% of haemangiomas may not respond.

1.18 CYSTIC HYGROMA

SCENARIO (no clinical photograph)	You are asked to see an 18 month-old child with a history of neck swelling since birth. 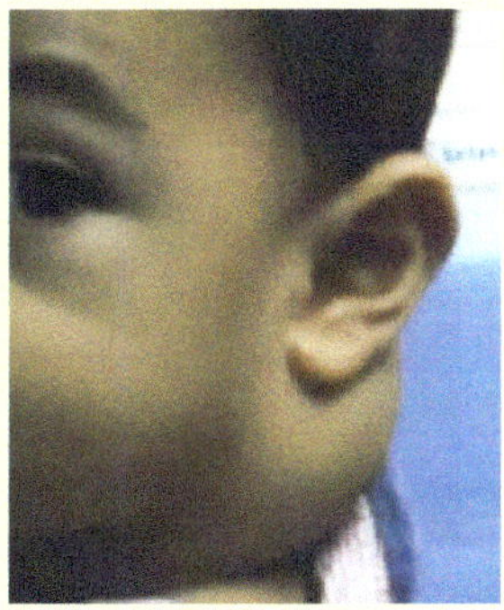

Introductory question	Answer
What is your differential diagnosis?	• Cervical cystic hygroma • Haemangioma • Teratoma • Simple cyst • Branchial cyst • Cervical lymphadenopathy secondary to e.g. atypical mycobacteria
Competency	**Answer**

question(s)	
How might they present and how would you manage this child?	• Typically present with soft, smooth, transilluminating, compressible, painless swelling in the posterior triangle of the neck. • Airway obstruction is possible • Microcystic oral disease may present with acute infection and bleeding Management is led by whether the disease is microcystic and macrocystic, whether it impacts or will impact on function and whether a staged approach is appropriate. MR imaging can provide a radiological diagnosis and stage the disease. Only 5% of such lesions spontaneously involve. The two treatment options are 1. Intra-lesional sclerotherapy – no consensus on best therapy. Requires ultrasound guided aspiration and injection under GA with acute inflammatory response needing to be covered with anti-inflammatories or occasionally elective intubation. 2. Open excision – aim to debulk macrocystic disease. Oral, pharyngeal or laryngeal disease may be treated with surface coblation.
Advanced question(s)	**Answer**
Describe a staging	***De Seres Classification (STAGE – LOCATION)***

system for cervico-facial cystic hygroma.	I Unilateral infrahyoid II Unilateral suprahyoid III Unilateral, supra and infrahyoid IV Bilateral suprahyoid V Bilateral supra and infrahyoid ***Giguere Classification*** • Macrocystic – cystic spaces at least 2cm or more • Microcystic – cystic spaces less than 2cm • Mixed
Give an example of a sclerosant used for intra-lesional sclerotherpy and give alternatives.	All sclerosants work by the same principle of provoking an inflammatory thus causing fibrosis and obliterating cystic spaces OK-432, (Picibanil) • Inactive strain of Group A Streptococcus pyogenes. Unique challenge is highly variable availability. • This is not licensed in the UK. Doxycycline • 10mg/ml by ultrasound guided injection under GA. Maximum suggested dose of 100mg for term children ≤12months and 200mg if >12months. Unique side-effects include possible hypoglycaemia and macrolide hypersensitivity.

1.19 THYROGLOSSAL DUCT CYST

Clinical photograph	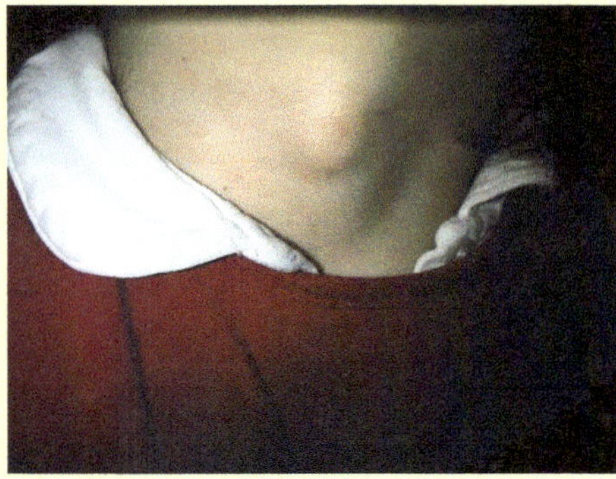

Introductory question	**Answer**
What is the differential diagnosis?	• Thyroglossal duct cyst (TGDC) • Midline dermoid cyst • Sebaceous cyst • Midline branchial cleft cyst • Lymph node
Competency question(s)	**Answer**
What clinical test might assist in diagnosis?	• TGDC will elevate on both swallowing and tongue protrusion. • TGDC represents the failure of

Explain how the embryology of thyroglossal duct cyst informs the operative management.	obliteration of the developmental tract that the thyroid tissue makes from its origin at the foramen caecum of the tongue (junction of the anterior 2/3 and posterior 1/3). • Complete excision of the TGDC should include the descending tract from the tongue base across the midline of the hyoid bone. This forms the embryological basis of the Sistrunk procedure. • Thyroid tissue within the TGDC may represent the only functioning thyroid tissue. This may be established by pre-operative cervical us/s to minimise the risk of removing the only functioning thyroid tissue.
Advanced question(s)	**Answer**
What are the main complications of this procedure and how might these be minimised?	• Procedure specific complications are accidental pharyngostomy, hypoglossal nerve injury and TGDC recurrence. • Pharyngostomy may be minimised by careful dissection on the deep surface of the TGDC. CN12 injury is minimised by avoiding the lateral cornu of the hyoid. TDGC recurrence may be further improved by performing an en-bloc resection of the central compartment tissue either side of the TGDC tract up to the hyoid bone and tongue base.

1.20 LINGUAL THYROID

CLINICAL PHOTOGRAPH	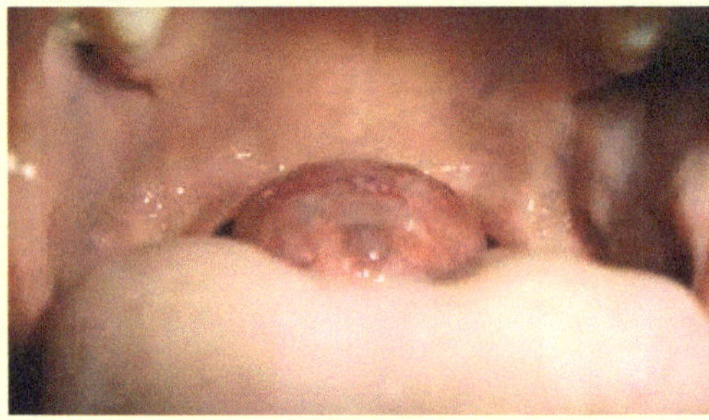

Introductory question	Answer
What is the differential diagnosis?	• Lingual thyroid • Thyroglossal duct cyst • Midline branchial cleft cyst • Lymphangioma • Dermoid cyst • Minor salivary gland tumour • Tongue base tumour
Competency question(s)	**Answer**
What investigations	• Technetium Tc-99m sodium thyroid scan. This will confirm the nature of the

could you perform to confirm the diagnosis? How would you manage this patient?	swelling and establish the presence of functioning thyroid tissue elsewhere. In 75% cases the ectopic thyroid tissue represents the only functioning thyroid tissue in the body. • Most ectopic tissue is asymptomatic but may increase in size and become symptomatic during puberty and pregnancy. It is four times more common in females. They may bleed, and malignant transformation has been reported. • In symptomatic older patients unfit for complete resection partial trans-oral ablation is suggested. Radioactive iodine ablation has also been used. • In younger patients with a consequently greater risk of malignant transformation complete resection is advised. If possible trans-orally or otherwise by trans-cervical pharyngostomy and a covering tracheostomy. Post-operative T4 replacement may be given to suppress ectopic thyroid tissue recurrence.
Advanced question(s)	**Answer**
What are the main sites of ectopic thyroid tissue?	• Lingual • Sublingual • Pre-tracheal • Mediastinal

1.21 CONGENITAL MIDLINE NASAL MASS

SCENARIO (clinical photograph)	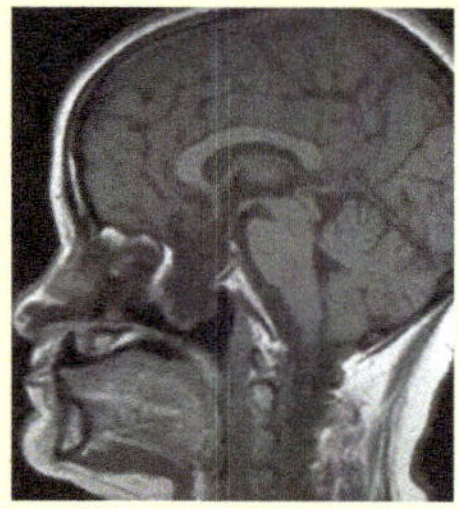 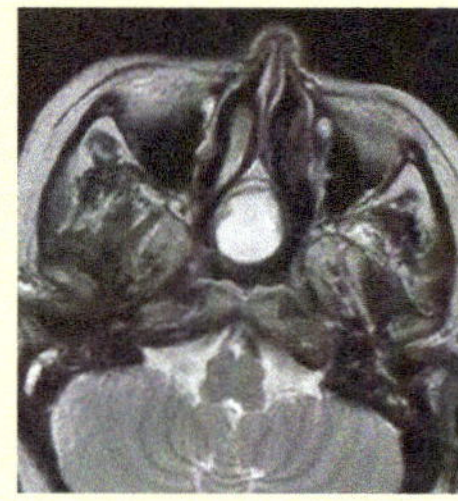

Introductory question	Answer
Describe what you see in the MR Images.	• T1 weighted image showing a midline line nasal lesion communicating with the third ventricle of the brain and T2 weighted image of the same lesion; the most likely diagnosis is a third ventricular encephalocele.
What is the differential diagnosis for midline nasal mass?	• Nasal glioma • Nasal dermoid • Encephalocele • Meningoencephalocele
Competency question(s)	**Answer**
How would	• **History** – Increase in size of the lesion on

manage this patient?	crying or straining. Previous meningitis. Vaccination history. • **Examination** – nasal endoscopic examination. Furstenberg sign - compression of the ipsilateral jugular vein leads to an increase in size of the mass. • **Investigation** – combined CT and MR imaging to determine the presence and nature of intra-cranial extension. • **Treatment** – early planned surgery is advised due to risk of meningitis in the presence of cyst infection and intra-cranial tract extension.
Advanced question(s)	**Answer**
A MRI was performed and demonstrates a cystic lesion with no intracranial extension. Describe your surgical approach.	• No biopsy to be performed • I would use a transverse or lateral rhinotomy incision. If the lesion extended into the lower half of the nose an open rhinoplasty approach may be used. • If intra-nasal components are present they may be removed with a combined endoscopic resection. • Any intra-cranial extension necessitates the assistance of an anterior skull-base surgeon who may use a sub-frontal craniotomy for access and dural repair.

1.22 CLEFT LIP AND PALATE

CLINICAL PHOTO	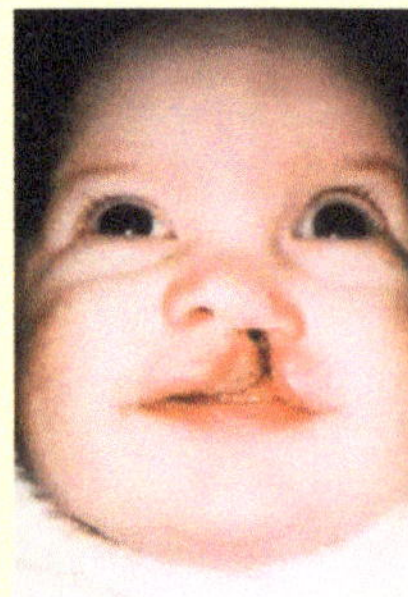

Introductory question	Answer
What is the diagnosis?	• Unilateral cleft lip • Would need to perform oral examination to determine extent and palatal integrity.
Competency question(s)	**Answer**
Describe a classification system for clefts and a schedule of treatment justifying your answer.	• Clefting may be of the lip, palate or combined (CLAP). • Primary palatal clefting is anterior to the incisive foramen and can include the alveolus. Secondary palatal cleft are posterior to incisive foramen and may

	involve the soft palate. • Veau classification of palatal cleft: Class 1 – isolated soft palate Class 2 – isolated hard palate Class 3 - unilateral CLAP Class 4 – bilateral CLAP • Management requires a multidisciplinary approach including speech and language therapist, orthodontist, facial plastic and cleft surgeon. • Infancy – cleft lip repair once 10weeks or 10 pounds, to aid oral feeding • Toddler – cleft palate repair at 10months to aid phonation • Late childhood – alveolar bone grafting at 12years +/- dental implant • Early adulthood – midfacial advancement and rhinoplasty options.
Advanced question(s)	**Answer**
Describe the clinical features of submucosal clefting and its relevance to the ENT surgeon.	• Failure of midline fusion of soft palate musculature. Typically associated with a bifid uvula and midline notching of the free border of the hard palate. • Resulting weakness in the Eustachian tube dilators increases the tendency to recurrent OME. • Adenoidectomy may result in

	velopharyngeal insufficiency (VPI) • Children with suspected submucosal cleft are best assessed prior to adenoidectomy by the cleft MDT. Alternatively suction diathermy adenoidectomy may be undertaken leaving a band of tissue against which the soft palate may approximate to minimise the risk of permanent VPI.

1.23 CONGENITAL CHOLESTEATOMA

SCENARIO (and clinical photograph)	You are asked to see a 10yrs-old child who is complaining of unilateral hearing loss. On Otoscopy a white mass is seen behind the tympanic membrane. 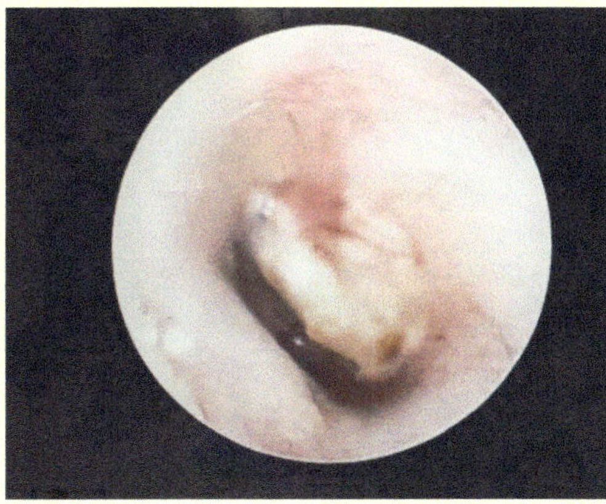

Introductory question	Answer
What is the most likely clinical diagnosis?	Congenital cholesteatoma.
Competency question(s)	**Answer**

What are the requirements for a diagnosis of congenital cholesteatoma? How does the location of congenital cholesteatoma differ from primary acquired cholesteatoma.	• ***The Derlacki and Clemis criteria require***: 1. White mass medial to an intact TM 2. Normal *pars tensa* and *pars flacida* 3. No previous ear surgery, otorrhoea or perforation • Congenital cholesteatoma typically begins in the antero-superior mesotympanum and is described to be more extensive on presentation but no more likely to recur if completely excised.
Advanced question(s)	**Answer**
Describe how the aetiology of congenital cholesteatoma differs from primary acquired cholesteatoma.	Several theories have been proposed to explain the congenital cholesteatoma. These include: 1. Persistence of epidermal rest cells in the middle ear. 2. Epithelial cells present in the amniotic fluid may enter the middle ear cleft and subsequently grow into a cholesteatoma. Theories for acquired cholesteatoma include: 1. Immigration 2. Retraction 3. hyperplasia due to chronic inflammation

	4. Metaplasia due to vit deficiency 5. Implantation For further details see Persaud *et al* 2007 "An evidence-based review of the aetiopathogenic theories of congenital and acquired cholesteatoma." *Journal Laryngology Otology. 121 (11):1013-1019.*

1.24 WAARDENBURG SYNDROME

Clinical photograph	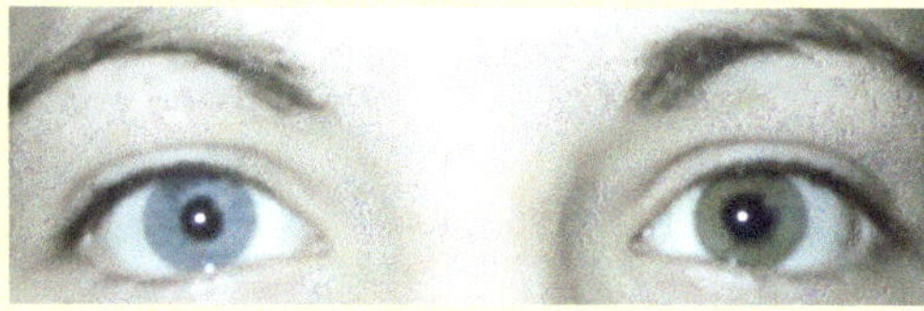

Introductory question	Answer
What is the diagnosis?	• Waardenburg syndrome – auditory-pigmentary syndrome.
Competency question(s)	**Answer**
List the syndromic features of Waardenburg syndrome.	• Clinical diagnosis requires 2 major criteria or 1 major and 2 minor • **Major** – dystopia canthorum, white forelock, heterochromia iridium, congenital SNHL, affected first degree relative • **Minor** – high and broad nasal root, hypoplastic nasal alae, medial eyebrow flare, skin hypopigmentation, premature greying of hair • **Type 1** – with dystopia canthorum

	• **Type 2** – without dystopia canthorum • **Type 3** – as for type 1 plus musculoskeletal abnormality • **Type 4** – as for type 2 plus Hirschprung's disease.
Advanced question(s)	**Answer**
What is the pattern of inheritance of the various subtypes?	• Type 1/2/3 are inherited in an autosomal dominant fashion. • Type 4 is inherited in an autosomal recessive fashion. • Type 1/3 – heterozygous haploinsufficiency from PAX3 mutation • Type 2 – MITF mutation. • Type 4 – homozygous mutation in EDN3 (endothelin 3) or endothelin receptor B (EDNRB).

1.25 RANULA

SCENARIO (clinical photograph)	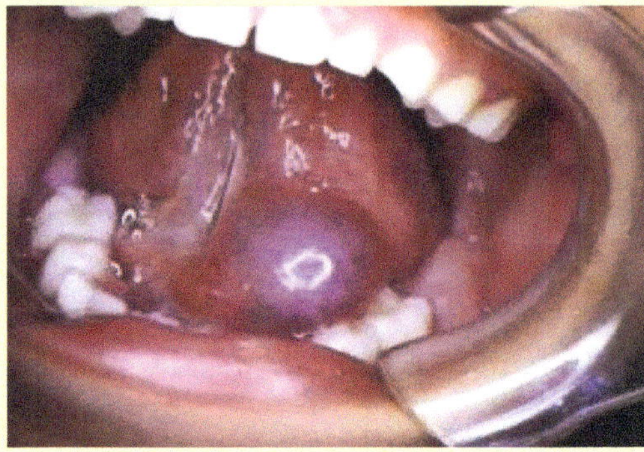

Introductory question	Answer
What is the differential diagnosis?	• Extravasation mucocele (ranula) • Lymphangioma • Dermoid cyst • Supra-hyoid thyroglossal duct cyst • Ectopic thyroid
Competency question(s)	**Answer**
How would you manage this patient?	• The diagnosis is clinical but may be aided by aspiration of mucus from the ranula and a staging MRI if there is significant

	cervical extension. • If symptomatic the pseudo-cyst can be treated by intra-lesional sclerosant but the most effective therapy is complete excision of the cyst and associated causative salivary gland – typically the sublingual. • Large ranula may 'descend' through the floor of mouth musculature into the neck. Such lesions often require intra-operative decompression to facilitate excision.
Advanced question(s)	**Answer**
Please explain why ranula formation may complicate Wharton's duct repositioning.	• The sublingual gland empties into several small ducts (ducts of Rivinus) which unite to form the duct of Bartholin which in turn drains onto the submandibular duct. Repositioning surgery may injure Bartholin's duct leading to ranula formation. • The risk of ranula formation may be minimised by resecting the sublingual gland when repositioning Wharton's duct.

1.26 CERVICAL LYMPHADENOPATHY

SCENARIO	GP referral: Please could you see this 4 year old boy with a lump behind right angle of jaw/upper neck 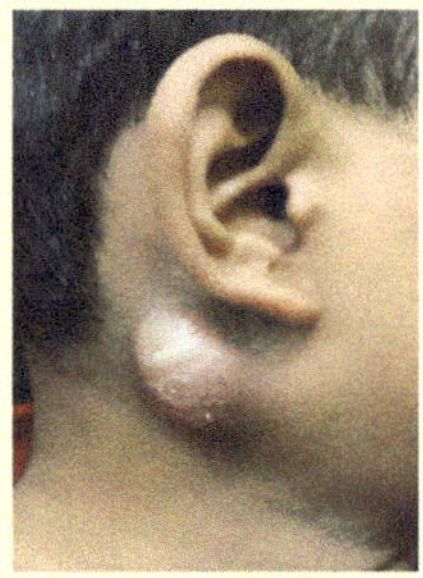

Introductory question	**Answer**
Describe the clinical photograph.	• This is a clinical photograph showing a swelling in level II of the neck of a child.
Competency question(s)	**Answer**
What points are you going to cover in the history and what are you going to look for on	• ***History***: duration, change in size, URTI, Child well, skin conditions scalp, weight loss, night sweats • ***Examination:*** Size, site, shape, skin over lump, temperature, tenderness,

<table>
<tr><td>examining him?

What would make you reassure and discharge a child with lymphadenopathy at first appointment?

What would make you list such a child for excision biopsy at first appointment? Are there any tests you would want pre-op?

If you are not discharging or listing the child what are you going to do?

And what do you do at the next appointment?</td><td>transillumination, consistency, attachment, mobility, pulsatility, fixed, reducible, irreducible, additional lumps. Ears nose & throat examination, Axillae or groin lymphadenopathy , hepatosplenomegally.

• Discharge: History of association URTI, Fluctuating in size, Soft, small (<2cm), mobile nodes, Instruct to return if nodes get progressively bigger

• List for excision: Supraclavicular LN, Node >3cm, History of malignancy, Generalised lymphadenopathy, Hepatosplenomegally

• Fever, weight loss night sweats

• Tests pre-op FBC, CXR (to exclude mediastinial lymph nodes)

• Neither discharge nor excise; CXR, FBC, Serology for Bartonella, EBV, CMV, toxoplasma and Brucellosis and HIV testings. Ultrasound Neck

• Then next appointment...

– If serology positive (10%)– Discharge

– If negative and lump same or bigger – List for excision

– If negative and lump smaller - Discharge</td></tr>
<tr><td>Advanced question(s)</td><td>Answer</td></tr>
<tr><td>What do you know about</td><td>• Malignant proliferation of the lymphoid system associated with B-symptoms:</td></tr>
</table>

lymphoma?	weight loss, night sweats and fevers. • May be Hodgkin's or non-Hodgkin's lymphoma depending on the presence of Reed-Sternberg cells. • 4 subtypes of Hodgkin's lymphoma (i) Nodular sclerosing (ii) Mixed Cellularity (iii) Lymphocyte predominant and (iv) Lymphocyte depleted • Diagnosis by lymph node biopsy. • Staging: CT Chest and abdomen, bone marrow biopsy, Stage 1 - Confined to single lymph node region. Stage 2 – Involvement of 2 or more regions on same side of diaphragm. Stage 3 – Involvement of nodes on both sides of the diaphragm. Stage 4 – Spread beyond the lymph nodes.

1.27 TRAUMATIC PERFORATION OF TYMPANIC MEMBRANE AND NON-ACCIDENTAL INJURY (NAI)

SCENARIO	A 5 year old boy is brought to the Emergency Department (ED) by his parents with a bleeding, bruised and swollen right ear. His Mother stated that he fell onto that side 5 days ago and it has only now started bleeding and become swollen. When the ED registrar assessed the child, his Father stated that he had been hit in the ear at school yesterday. On examination, you notice a fresh bruise over his right pinna and mastoid area and an older bruise around his left eye. There is dried blood at his meatus. Dad states that the eye bruise had happened at school. The child looks scared and does not talk to you.

Introductory question	Answer
What is your differential diagnosis?	• Blunt ear trauma • Pinna Haematoma • Underlying coagulopathy • Balance disorder leading to falls • Otitis Media with perforation

	• Non-accidental injury (NAI)
Competency question(s)	**Answer**
This is what is seen on Otoscopy. Describe what you see and explain your diagnosis. 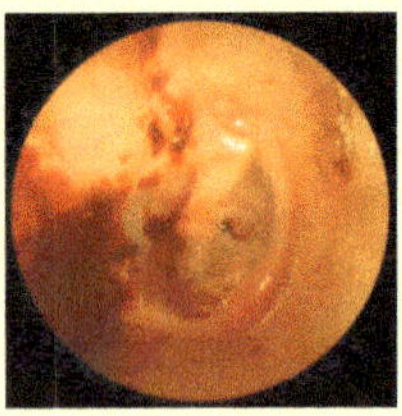	• This an otoscopic image showing a right tympanic membrane with an anterior perforation. There is a haematoma of the posterior wall of the ear canal and blood crusts in the canal. This would be consistent with a spontaneous or traumatic perforation. In the absence of any history of infection, and in the presence of external bruising, a traumatic perforation by non-accidental injury would be the most likely diagnosis. • A fall onto this ear five days ago, causing this amount of trauma would be unlikely. The bleeding would have occurred immediately after the injury and the bruising and swelling would have come on within an hour – not five days later. • A blow to that ear the day previously may be a plausible explanation, however it would have needed to be a blow of considerable force to cause a perforation, and the school are likely to have a record of this. • The major alarming factor is the presence of multiple injuries of different ages. • The inconsistency and implausibility of the stories concerning the injuries are also an alerting factor, as are delayed presentations.

	• A quiet child who refuses to speak, or the so called "frozen watchfulness" in a post-lingual child are also signs to be aware of.
Advanced question(s)	**Answer**
How would you manage this case?	• In line with the GMC document "Good Medical Practice", it is the duty of all doctors to protect Children and Young People and act on any concerns they have about the safety or welfare of a child or young person. • You must read the GMC guidance on protecting Children and Young people. • It is the duty of every doctor working with, or coming into contact with children, to be aware of their local child protection procedures. • If I am concerned about NAI, I would inform the the Responsible Officer of the Child Protection Team at the hospital; this is usually a paediatric doctor. The team will carry out the necessary assessment and then liaise with the appropriate agency, such as your local authority children's services, the NSPCC or the police. • If there is serious concern, admit the child to hospital to allow time to contact local child protection services and enlist their expertise. • It is important to explore all possibilities of diagnosis including NAI, as rare causes

	can sometimes be missed. • It is important to make sure that the clinical needs of the child are met and not overshadowed by the child protection concerns. In this case consider topical antibiotics and aural toilet to remove crusts.

1.28 CAUSTIC INGESTION AND NON-ACCIDENTAL INJURY

SCENARIO **(no clinical photograph)**	You are asked to see a 10 month old in A+E who was brought by her mother with reluctance to drink having been alone in the kitchen. She is apyrexial but drooling with ulceration to chin and lips.

Introductory question	Answer
What is your differential diagnosis?	• Caustic ingestion +/- NAI neglect • Herpes stomatitis • Kawasaki disease
Competency question(s)	**Answer**
How would you manage this patient?	• **History** – What may have been ingested, when, volume and has the bottle been recovered. Alkali results in a deeper liquefactive necrosis than the coagulative necrosis of acids. • **Examination** – Evidence of airway compromise and staging of injury. Inspect for signs of NAI eg injury out of keeping with a child of that age. • **Investigations** – In conjunction with a

	paediatrician blood taken for paracetamol and salicylate levels. • **Treatment** – If airway compromise present child will likely need to be intubated in theatre. If not emergent an upper endoscopy should be carried out within 48hrs to stage extent and depth of injury. Any ulcerative processes require prophylactic antibiotics, PPI +/- corticosteroids. Nasogastric tube insertion and parenteral nutrition should be considered. • **Follow-up** – be observant for complications including bleeding, perforation/sepsis and stricture formation.
Advanced question(s)	**Answer**
What would you do?	• These are signs consistent with physical abuse or potential neglect. • I would liaise with a paediatrician specialising in child protection who in turn should liaise with the statutory child protection authority. I would ensure that the child remains in a place of safety until this is achieved and that the nursing staff are aware of these concerns. • I would take a full social history and consider the need to protect any siblings at home from abuse. • Consider the need for support and protection of other family members within a multi-agency team framework.

1.29 JUVENILE NASOPHARYNGEAL ANGIOFIBROMA (JNA)

SCENARIO (no clinical photograph)	A 14 year old boy presents to your outpatient clinic with progressively worsening intermittent right-sided epistaxis.

Introductory question	Answer
What would you specifically look for in the history and on examination, and what is your differential diagnosis?	• Easily bruises • Family history of bleeding disorders • Intranasal prominent vessel or old bleeding point • Unilateral intranasal lesion • Idiopathic epistaxis • Digital trauma • Allergic rhinitis • Bleeding disorder • Pyogenic granuloma • Juvenile nasopharyngeal angiofibroma (JNA)
Competency question(s)	**Answer**

After seeing a right-sided intranasal polypoidal lesion, how would you go on to investigate this case? CT imaging reports a likely JNA with anterior bowing of the posterior maxillary sinus wall. What is the name of this sign and its other feature?	**DO NOT BIOPSY!** **Differential** • JNA • Antrochoanal polyp • Pyogenic granuloma **Investigations** • CT/CTA, MRI/MRA or Carotid angiography (looking specifically at ascending pharyngeal or sphenopalatine arteries) • Holman-Miller sign – also includes posterior bowing of the pterygoid plate.

Advanced question(s)	Answer
How would you classify a JNA and what are the treatment options?	<u>Fisch Classification</u> I – limited to nasal cavity II – into sinuses or pterygomaxillary fossa (bony destruction) III – into infratemporal fossa or parasellar IV – into cavernous sinus, optic chiasm, pituitary <u>Treatment</u> • Embolise prior to surgery • Surgery 1) Endoscopic (if small) 2) Transpalatal (junction of hard/soft palate – rarely due to disruption of the growth plate) 3) Transantral (Caldwell-Luc) 4) Combined lateral rhinotomy and transnasal 5) Maxillary swing 6) Craniofacial resection (if cribiform plate involved) • Recurrence reduced by drilling basi-sphenoid

1.30 AIRWAY FOREIGN BODY

SCENARIO **(FOLLOWED BY A CLINICAL PHOTOGRAPH)**	An otherwise healthy 4 year old boy has been brought to Accident and Emergency by his anxious parents. He had been playing in the loft when they found him choking and coughing. He now appears to be well and does not have any acute airway problems.

Introductory question	Answer
What is going through your mind and what would you do?	• Based on the history and clinical presentation, this is an emergency situation with a possible foreign body in the aerodigestive tract
Competency question(s)	**Answer**
What would you do?	• I would go to see the child and family, staying calm and in control of the situation. • Quickly assess Airway, Breathing and Circulation • Take a targeted history – focusing of the incident, ie witnessed choking episode, vomiting, cyanosis neck trauma etc.

Ok. Here is the chest xray. Describe what you see. 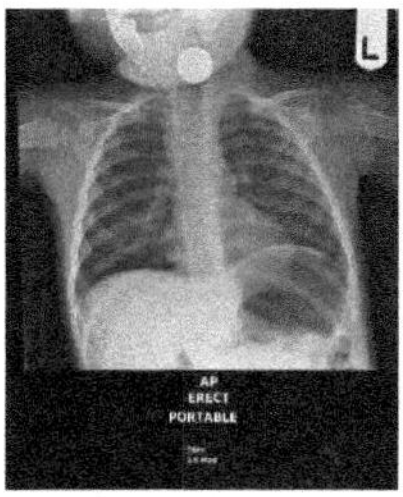 What will you do next?	• I would check for stridor, stertor, drooling, dysphagia and dyspnoea • Then I would consider requesting a chest x-ray • This is a portable erect AP chest x-ray showing a radiolucent object resembling a coin in the upper aerodigestive tract • I would also like to see a lateral view to assess if the FB is in the oesophagus, airway or in-between (intra-thoracic) • Inform the senior anaesthetist and paediatrician. Consider informing the senior emergency theatre coordinator about the case and to identify appropriate surgical instruments required (e.g. forceps, rigid endoscopes, paediatric tracehoestomy tubes etc.) • Do the above but ask for the senior anaesthetist, A&E consultant to be present. • Consider transferring the child to Majors or Resus. • Consider giving the child some Heliox (Mixture of helium and oxygen. The composition has a lower density than room air, thus making breathing easier in cases or airway obstruction.) • This child needs to go to theatre to have this foreign body removed. • Speak to the family and seek informed, signed consent.

	• If you had informed the other health-care professionals earlier, transfer to theatre may be more expeditious.
Advanced question(s)	**Answer**
What would you do if you were in a district general hospital and there was no paediatric anaesthetic cover?	• This is a clinical problem and the child should be kept in a calm, reassuring environment with his parents. You should contact your hub-and-spoke paediatric ENT unit urgently to discuss. They may either send out a retrieval team or a complete surgical team to remove the foreign body in theatre.
Name and describe the components in this picture. 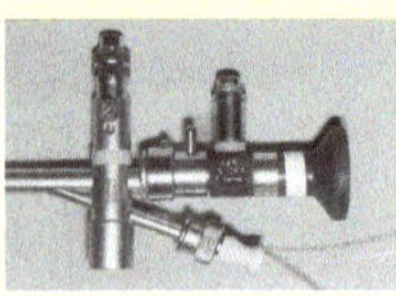	• Ventilating bronchoscope, locking mechanism for endoscope, suction portal, adaptor for ventilation circuit, extension collar on the bronchoscope (to fit with the endoscope) light prism

1.31 SLEEP DISORDERED BREATHING IN A CHILD

SCENARIO **(no clinical photograph)**	A GP refers you a 3 year old boy with snoring and intermittent episodes of cessation of breathing. The GP is concerned about the child sleep disordered breathing, in particular obstructive sleep apnoea.

Introductory question	Answer
What do you understand by sleep disordered breathing?	A spectrum of conditions ranging from 1. Snoring (normal blood gases) 2. Upper airway resistant syndrome (paradoxical and out of phase breathing, increased pulse transit time) 3. Obstructive hypoventilation (mild hypercapnia) 4. Obstructive sleep apnoa (hypercapnia and hypoxia)
Competency question(s)	**Answer**
How would you assess the child in clinic?	**History** *1.* ***Nocturnal***: snoring, number of episodes of cessations of breathing, sweating, bed wetting, sword swallowing position,

When would you refer a child for respiratory investigations such as polysomnography or to a tertiary paediatric centre?	restless sleep, frequent awaking. 2. ***Diurnal***: hyperactive, poor concentration, swallowing issues, mouth breathing. **Full ENT Examination** (syndromic, nasal obstruction, mouth breathing, large tongue, adenoidal face, OME). **Investigations** (consider overnight pulse oximetry or full sleep study if child is syndromic or failure to thrive is present. • Diagnosis of OSA is unclear • Age under 2 yrs • Weight under 15kg • Down • Cerebral palsy • Hypotonia/Neuromuscular disorders • Craniofacial abnormalities • Mucopolysaccharidosis • Obesity • Significant co-morbidity • Residual symptoms after adequate adenotonsillectomy
Advanced question(s)	**Answer**
Why might you need a HDU bed in a tertiary referral centre?	• Pulmonary oedema may occur post operatively, when the cause for the obstruction (eg adenotonsillar hypertrophy) has been removed. o PEEP may be required in a HDU setting.

CHAPTER 2

Rhinology and Facial Plastics

2.1 ANOSMIA

SCENARIO **(followed by radiological images)**	A 55 year old male chef complains of inability to detect odours. He has no significant past medical history and is otherwise fit and well.

Introductory question	**Answer**
How would you manage this patient in clinic?	• This patient may be suffering from anosmia and therefore I would start by taking a targeted history on the aetiology of the condition, i.e. conductive and sensorineural causes of Anosmia • I would then proceed to examine the nose with a rigid nasendoscope paying particular attention to the olfactory cleft areas. • If no obvious cause is found, I would proceed to investigate with a University

	of Pennsylvania Smell Investigation Test (UPSIT) or other smell test and maybe a MRI brain.
Competency question(s)	**Answer**
Here are the patient's MRI brain scans. Tell me what they show? 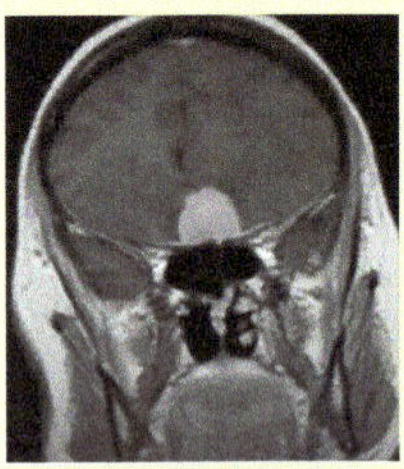 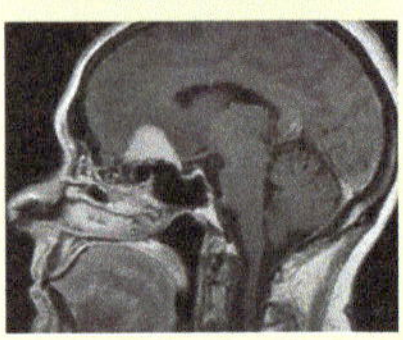 How would you counsel this patient?	• These are T1 contrast-enhanced MRI coronal and saggital sections showing a lesion in the olfactory region of the brain. • The lesion has a broad base and bilateral dural tails; these are features consistent with a meningioma. • Such lesion can account for the patient inability to detect odours (anosmia). • Refer to a neurosurgeon for management of the meningioma • Fit smoke alarms • Change gas cooker to electric as patient is unable to smell gas leak • Document and be aware of sell-by and use-by date on foods
Advanced question(s)	**Answer**
What score on UPSIT would you expect from a laryngectomy	Due to lack of air flow, laryngectomy patients become anosmic and therefore would score around 10/40. This is because the probability of getting a correct answer is 1 in 4 and

patient and do you think that it is different in a malingerer?	patients are told to guess if they don't know. A malingerer will score approximately 0-5/40.

2.2 CSF RHINORHOEA

SCENARIO (no clinical photograph)	You are asked to see a 45year-old overweight woman with persistent clear unilateral nasal discharge.

Introductory question	Answer
What is your differential diagnosis?	• Cerebrospinal Fluid (CSF) rhinorrhoea • Vasomotor rhinitis • Gustatory rhinitis • Allergic rhinitis
Competency question(s)	**Answer**
Assuming you suspect CSF rhinorrhoea, how would you manage the case?	• **History** –focused history for head trauma, nasal surgery and symptoms of meningism. • **Examination** – observe leak with head in dependent position or by placement of pledgets to collect sample • **Investigations –** Tau protein analysis of >0.5ml of fluid to confirm diagnosis; if positive and atraumatic - localise source of leak by CT of skull-base to include temporal bone. (Tegmen or petrous apex

	leak with fluid filling middle ear and tracking down the Eustachian tube can present with rhinorrhoea). Also T2 weighted MRI (where CSF signal is high). Pre-operative intra-thecal fluorosceine may be used to further localise. • **Treatment** – advise to seek medical attention if develop signs of meningeal irritation. If following head injury – head up bed rest, laxatives for 1/52. Surgery and lumbar drain if not settling. If atraumatic then surgical repair following localisation by endoscopic or open technique with neurosurgeon.
Advanced question(s)	**Answer**
What is Idiopathic Intracranial Hypertension and what is its relationship with CSF rhinorrhoea	• A syndrome of raised intracranial pressure (ICP) in the absence of hydrocephalus most often seen in the obese. Chronic raised ICP is suspected to lead to skull base remodelling which predisposes to CSF leak. May also lead to optic nerve atrophy. • Diagnosis is based on history, slit ventricles on CT and raised ICP on LP • May require temporary lumbar drain post-op to reduce risk of leak repair failure.

2.3 FUNGAL RHINOSINUSITIS

SCENARIO **(and IMAGING)**	GP referral: Please could you kindly see this 42 year old lady with a history of recurrent episodes of sinusitis, occurring 4 times each winter, requiring antibiotics on each occasion and which is now causing her significant symptoms. A CT scan was organised and here is a section. 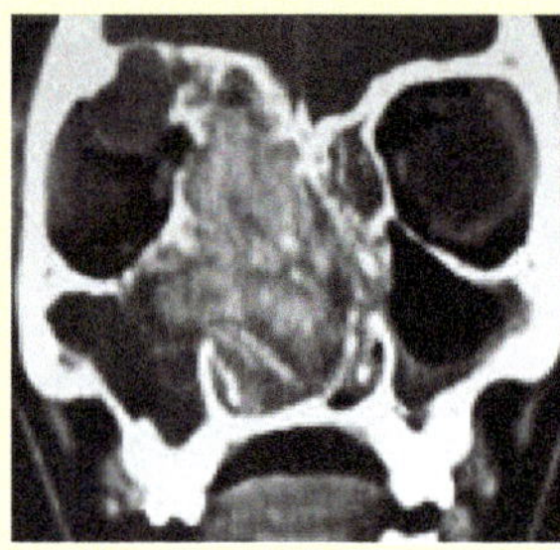

Introductory question	Answer
Describe the imaging.	• Coronal CT scan of the nose and paranasal sinuses, showing unilateral opacification of the right maxillary, ethmoid sinuses. Some irregularities and heterogeneity noted within the substance of the maxillary sinus. There is a large expansive mass within the right side of the nose leading to extensive

	bony remodelling. There appears to be an extension of the lesion into the right orbit with a possible mucocele.
Competency question(s)	**Answer**
What is the differential diagnosis?	**Differential:** • Acute on chronic rhinosinusitis • Recurrent acute rhinosinusitis • Fungal rhinosinusitis • Antrochoanal polyp/Nasal polyposis • Inverted papilloma • Dental abscess • Neoplastic lesion (although in this scan the opacification extends to involve the anterior and posterior ethmoid sinuses as well)
How do you diagnose fungal sinusitis?	***Diagnosis based on Bent & Kuhn diagnostic. criteria (5 major)*** 1. Atopy (on history or serology to fungal antigen or allergy testing) 2. Nasal polyposis 3. Characteristic CT scan findings 4. Positive fungal smear 5. Allergic mucin
Do you know of any classification of fungal	NB. In addition there are 6 minor criteria (asthma, unilateral predominance, bone erosion on radiography, fungal culture,

sinusitis?	charcot leiden crystals, eosinophilia). In practice, you may also add MRI scan findings to this list owing to the well described ferromagnetic properties of fungi. Some of these criteria are only diagnosed postoperatively however, hence their limitations for clinical diagnosis. **Classification** • Invasive (acute, such as mucormycosis vs chronic) • Non-invasive (fungal ball, Allegic fungal rhinosinusitis) **OR** • **Fungal Ball** – non-invasive, usually Aspergillus, typically unilateral maxillary sinus, may have unilateral proptosis/facial hypesthesia, Histo – Y-shaped hyphae, endoscopic removal • **Allergic** – fungal infection (Aspergillus, molds) leading to antigen for allergic response, rhinorrhoea/nasal congestion, RAST for fungus/molds, no invasion, endoscopic debridement, topical steroids +/- antifungals • **Acute Invasive (Mucormycosis)** – rapidly invades bone/soft tissue (necrosis)/vessels (thombus/infacts), Aspergillus/Mucor/Rhizopus, immunocompromised (DM, chemo, HIV, bone marrow transplant), 50% mortality with CNS/cavernous sinus involvement, Histo – T-shaped hyphae, Surgical debridement and Amphotericin B

	Chronic Invasive – Rare, indolent invasion of soft tissues (but otherwise similar to acute), surgical debridement and long term Amphotericin B and Itraconazole for 1 year
Advanced question(s)	**Answer**
What is the evidence that fungi are in fact causal to the symptoms of chronic rhinosinusitis? Do you treat with antifungals and what is the evidence that they are effective?	• Fungi have been shown to be almost ubiquitous in nasal samples – up to 97% (Ponikau, Mayo Clinic). However the type of sample (eg. Surface smear versus a washing) or whether PCR applied causes wide variations in yield. Also allergy identified to fungal antigen not always the type of fungus identified in the nasal sample, evidence collectively suggesting therefore that the fungus may be a commensal rather than a pathogen. *Antifungals:* Double-blind placebo and randomised controlled trials exist for both oral and topical antifungal agents compared against placebo controls. Some evidence exists that they are effective even in CRS patients.

2.4 HEREDITARY HAEMORRHAGIC TELANGECTASIA (HHT)

SCENARIO (clinical photographs of tongue and face of the same patient)	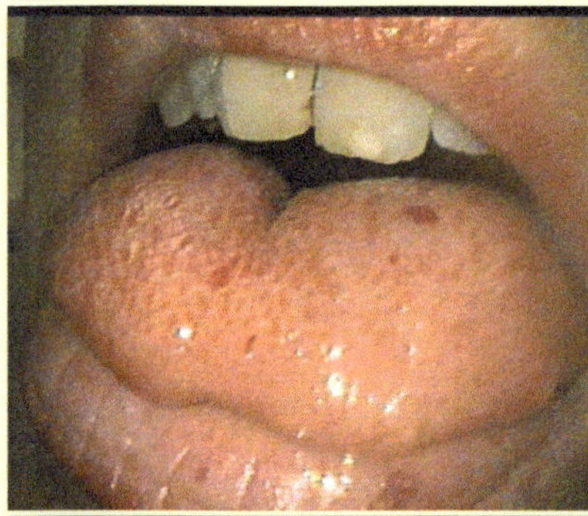 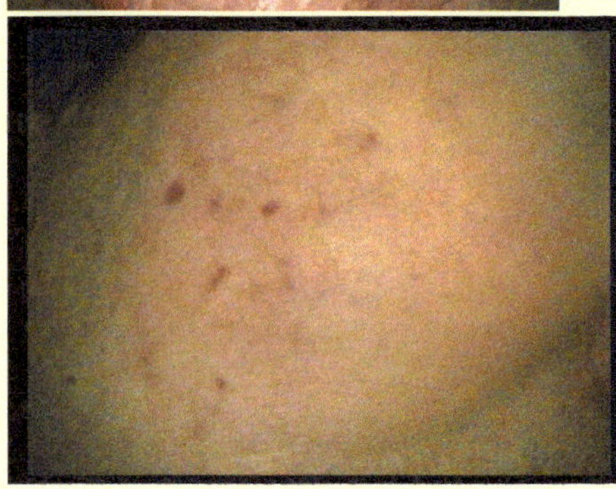

Introductory question	Answer
Look at the images and tell me is the	• Hereditary haemorrhagic telangiectasia (HHT) (aka Osler-Weber-Rendu syndrome) Differentials would include:

diagnosis.	• Capillary malformation-AVM syndrome • CREST syndrome • Hereditary benign telangiectasia • Bleeding disorders (ie. Von Willebrand disease) Diagnosis is based on 4 criteria: • Epistaxis (spontaneous and recurrent) • Telangiectasias (lips, oral cavity, fingers, nasal septum) • Internal Lesions (GI telangiectasia, pulmonary/hepatic/brain AVMs) • Family History (first degree relative with HHT) >2 – Definite >1 – Possible 0-1 - Unlikely
Competency question(s)	**Answer**
What is HHT? Tell me about the genetics of HHT.	• HHT is a genetic disorder of the blood vessel wall, characterized by abnormal blood vessel unable to contract. • Autosomal dominant (5 genetic types) • HHT1 (Chromosome 9q33-34) • HHT2 (Chromosome 12q11-14) • HHT3 (Chromosome 5q31 (unidentified gene)) • HHT4 (Chromosome 7p14 (unidentified gene)) • HHT and juvenile polyposis – MADH4

<table>
<tr>
<td>How would you manage this patient?
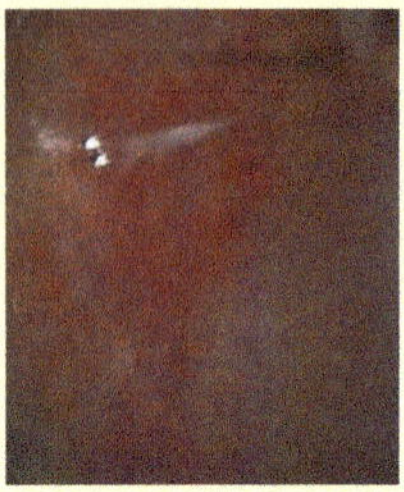
Figure 2.4a.Nasal mucosa of a HHT patient

What are the treatment options for a HHT patient presenting with recurrent chronic troublesome epistaxis.
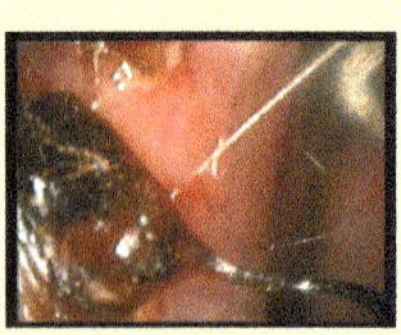
Figure 2.4b. Clots</td>
<td>(Chromosome 18q21)
• HHT1 – pulmonary and cerebral AVMs higher than HHT2 and oral/nasal mucosal telangectasias present earlier.
• HHT2 – Hepatic AVMs higher than in HHT1
• Take great care when examining such patients in clinic as even rigid nasendoscopy can trigger a significant epistaxis. Avoid unnecessary instrumentation where possible.
• Epistaxis is most common presentation, followed by bleeds anywhere in the GI tract, AVMs (pulmonary, liver, intracranial). Telangiectasia on finger tips.
History:
• spontaneous recurrent epistaxis. FH. Frequency of blood transfusions to assess severity.

Examination:
• Oral mucosal telangectasia
• Nasal mucosal telangectasia
• Conjunctival or retinal telangectasia
• Focal neurology in brain AVM
• Tachypnoea/cyanosis/clubbing/pulmonary bruit in pulmonary AVM
• Jaundice/hepatosplenomegaly/right upper quadrant bruit or thrill</td>
</tr>
</table>

in the nose of a HHT patient	• Signs of anaemia • nasal, oral and digital examination. **Investigations:** • FBC, Clotting • ABGs – low pO2 in right-to-left shunt • Imaging – CXR then CT or Transthoracic contrast echocardiogram (pulmonary AVM), MRI or CT (Brain AVM), MRI (Spinal AVM), Doppler ultrasound • Diagnose by FH, muco-cutaneous telangiectasia and screen for visceral AVM so genetic testing will identify causative gene in the proband in 80% of cases. Family risk may be assessed by linkage analysis. **Acute Treatment** • Avoid traumatic packing in acute episodes. Kaltostat soaked in adrenaline or dissolvable nasopore is preferred to abrasive merocel. Transanexnic acid is helpful in prevent fibrinolysis. **Chronic Treatment** • **Medical Treatment:** Coagulation therapy is often the quickest way to stop epistaxis, but there is some controversy as to the best way to do this. Many experts believe that laser coagulation therapy (KTP laser) is preferable to electric and chemical cautery because it causes less damage to the inside of the nose. However, some experts have reported good success with bipolar electric cautery. Regardless of the

	method used, it is important to have coagulation therapy by someone who has expertise in treatment of HHT patients. Most patients who undergo coagulation therapy see significant improvement for a period of time, but it usually needs to be repeated periodically. • Sprays and ointments containing oestrogen, bevacizumab (Avastin), and tranexamic acid have been used in small numbers of patients and are currently being studied in clinical trials. • Several small research studies have suggested that various oral therapies can help some patients for whom the local therapies (i.e. home moisturizing care and laser therapy) have not been successful. Oral contraceptive pills have been used the most, and while they do seem to help some patients, they have significant side effects. Drugs that affect either the formation of clots or vasculature are being investigated (i.e., estrogens, tamoxifen, n-acetylcysteine, bevzcizumab (Avastin), and others) to examine the effectiveness and safety of these drugs. • **Surgical Treatment:** Septodermoplasty, Youngs Procedure and KTP laser are surgical treatment options, but are usually only considered when epistaxis is severe, significantly affecting quality of life and coagulation therapy has repeatedly failed to help. Septodermoplasty replaces the thin lining of the nose with a split skin graft. It can significantly reduce or stop

	haemorrhages, often for two or more years. Daily care of the nose is required after septodermoplasty to keep the nose moist and clean. In Youngs procedure, the nostrils are surgically closed with local skin flaps. This therapy is quite effective but the downside is that taste and smell are affected. • **Embolization:** This procedure blocks an artery which, in most cases, stops severe epistaxes that have been unresponsive to other treatments. This procedure is usually only effective for 6-8 weeks as collateral vessels enlarge and lead to recurrence. This therapy for the nose should be used only on an emergency basis until more durable therapies can be started.

Advanced question(s)	Answer
What does LASER mean?	• **L**ight **A**mplification by the **S**timulation **E**mission of **R**adiation
What are the properties of the KTP laser that make it suitable for HHT treatment?	• ***KTP laser:*** wavelength of 532nm puts it in visible spectrum (Bright green laser light); wavelength short enough so can go down a flexible tube; 532nm wavelength means that it is preferentially absorbed by red blood cells and vessels. Acts by coagulating vessels. Tends not to damage normal mucosa/skin.
What is the key surgical step in septodermoplasty	• Leave the ***perichondrial layer intact*** because it is the source of blood supply to the skin graft.
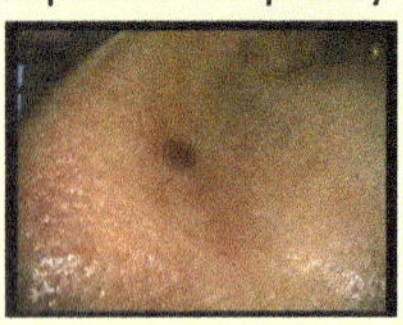 There is usually no bleeding from telangiectasias in the skin such as that seen on the nose. Why is that?	• Because of the protective squamous epithelial layer
What are the systemic complications of this condition and how might they be managed?	• Visceral AVM may present with GI/liver bleed, CNS/spinal CVA. Pulmonary AVM may lead to pulmonary haemorrhage or cerebral abscess. • Uncontrolled pulmonary AVM carry a mortality risk in pregnancy and should be referred for consideration of embolisation. • CNS AVM may be embolised but the role of CNS screening in the absence of symptoms is contentious and best made in an MDT.

2.5 ANTROCHOANAL POLYP

CLINICAL PHOTOGRAPH	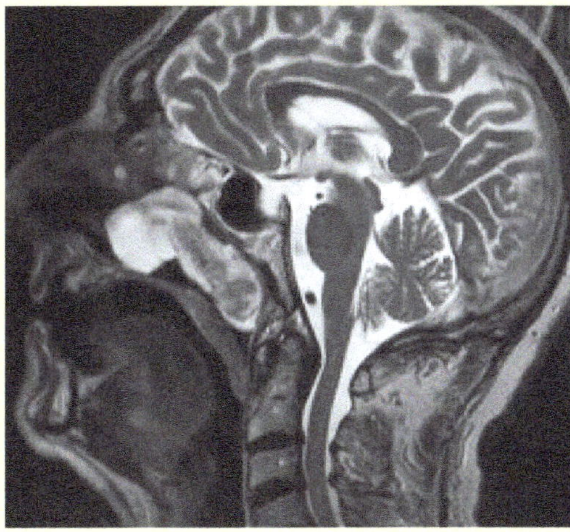

Introductory question	Answer
Tell me about this scan	• Saggital MRI T2 weighted showing a mix intensity lesion in the nasal cavity extending towards the choana • This is most likely to represent an antrochoanal polyp

Competency question(s)	Answer
What are the clinical features? What is the treatment?	<u>Clinical features</u>: • Unilateral, usually adolescent, young adults • Unilateral nasal obstruction • Unilateral nasal discharge • Headache (mostly unilateral) • Epistaxis • Sleep apnoea • Blocked nose • Difficulty in swallowing • OME • Endoscopic polypectomy with removal of the uncinate process • Recurrence may require a Caldwell Luc approach
Advanced question(s)	**Answer**
What is the pathogenesis of an antrochoanal polyp?	Theories: • May be due to faulty development of the maxillary sinus ostium (growth due to impediment to the venous return from the polyp) • Pressure drop next to a constriction causes a suction effect pulling the sinus

	mucosa into the nose • Mucopolysaccharide changes lead to polyp formation

2.6 SARCOIDOSIS

SCENARIO **(no clinical photograph)**	A 50 year old lady is under the respiratory team with worsening shortness of breath. She is referred to you by them because they have diagnosed a 'Bell's palsy'. She is also complaining of a painful red eye and cheek swelling.

Introductory question	Answer
Given the collection of symptoms, what is the most likely diagnosis?	• Sarcoidosis. The patient is demonstrating the signs of Uveoparotid fever (Heerfordt's disease)
Competency question(s)	**Answer**
What is sarcoidosis? What are the other presenting symptoms and complications of sarcoidosis?	• Systemic granulomatous disease. • Type IV hypersensitivity reaction, but antigen/ aetiology unknown. • Causes accumulation of mononuclear cells, leading to ***non-caseating granuloma*** formation followed by organ fibrosis (mainly affecting lungs), but is a

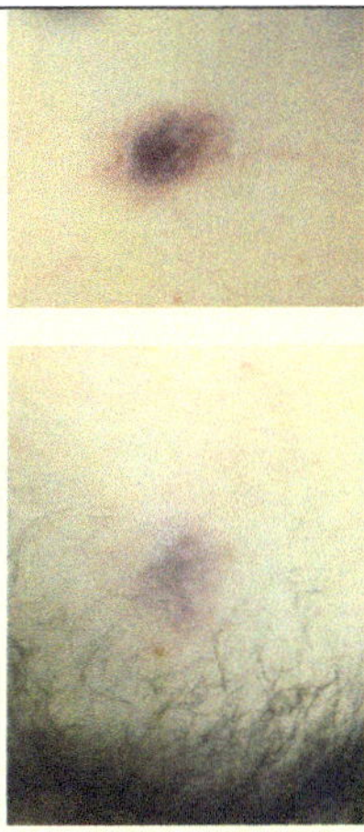 Sarcoidosis of the skin	multisystem disease. Symptoms/Complications • Can often be asymptomatic, being an incidental finding on a CXR (hilar lymphadenopathy) • Cough/SOB • Weight loss • Fever • Uveoparotid fever (uveitis, facial palsy, parotid swelling, fever, SNHL) • Cervical lymphadenopathy • Nasal crusting/mass/perforation • Supraglottic mass • Erythema nodosum • Subcutaneous nodules (Darier-Roussey nodules) • Liver dysfunction • Renal dysfunction • Splenomaegaly • Arrhythmias • Lytic or sclerotic bone lesions • Neuropathy
Advanced question(s)	**Answer**
How would you	• CXR – hilar lymphadenopathy

confirm the diagnosis of sarcoidosis?	• Raised serum ACE • Hypercalcaemia • Protein electrophoresis (hypergammaglobulinaemia) • Lung (or affected organ) biopsy
What is the histopathology involved in this condition?	• Accumulation of T-cells • Accumulation of mononuclear cells • Phagocytosis • Non-caseating granuloma formation • Fibrosis
What are the interventions for the ENT surgeon?	• Excision biopsy of cervical lymph node • Nasal septal biopsy • Managing sequelae of nasal septal perforation • Managing facial palsy/parotid involvement • Diagnosing and managing vocal cord palsy • Diagnostic rigid laryngoscopy +/- biopsy • Surgical excision of obstructing supraglottic lesions

2.7 SINONASAL TUMOUR

SCENARIO **FOLLOWED BY A CLINICAL PHOTOGRAPH**	A 55 year old man has been referred to you with a 6 months history of progressive left-sided nasal obstruction. More recently, he has been suffering with intermittent nasal discharge, scabbing and mild epistaxis.

Introductory question	Answer
What is your differential diagnosis? How would you assess this patient?	• **Benign:** Antrochoanal polyp, inverting papilloma, meningoencephaloceole • **Malignant:** Adenocarcinoma, squamous cell carcinoma, esthesioblastoma • **History:** Onset and severity of sinonasal symptoms, occupational history (hard word, toxic fumes) • **Examination:** In addition heck for cutaneous lesions, palpate for lymphadenopathy • Nasendoscopy
Competency question(s)	**Answer**
You were unable to pass the	• Radiological assessment e.g. CT and/or MRI of the paranasal sinuses, orbit, brain,

nasendoscope on the ipsilateral side which is completely occuded by a granular, fleshy, firm mass. On the contralateral nasal cavity, the septum was had a convex deviation, although the mucosa appeared healthy. What would you do next? Would you take a biopsy of the lump in clinic? How would you proceed with the management of this patient? Here are the MR images. Describe what you see. 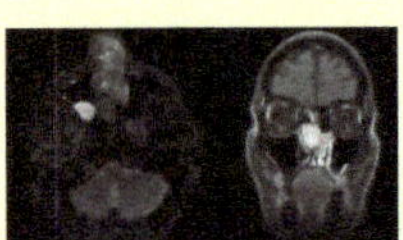	neck. • It is unwise to biopsy the lesion when intracranial extension is unknown (risk of CSF leak if the lesion was a meningoencephaloceole). Furthermore, the lesion may be highly vascular risking torrential epistaxis in the outpatients department. • Patients needs to have a biopsy of the lesion under GA for histological diagnosis and then discussion at the MDT. • Axial MRI scan demonstrating a left sided lesion occluding the entire nasal cavity with deviation of the septum to the right. • Coronal MRI scan more posteriorly showing that the mass does not appear to involve the skull base, posterior ethmoids and orbit.
Advanced	**Answer**

question(s)	
What do you think will be the decision at the MDT meeting? What are the surgical approaches?	• Major surgical excision, followed by post-operative radiotherapy. • Surgical approaches include external approach (e.g. lateral rhinotomy, midfacial degloving) or endoscopic resection (if this is the only option acceptable to the patient, he may need to be referred to a specialist endoscopic rhinologist).

2.8 OLFACTION

SCENARIO **(no clinical photograph)**	A 37 year old gentleman presents to your specialist rhinology clinic saying he has had a reduction in his sense of smell for the last 12 months.

Introductory question	**Answer**
What medical term would you use to assign to a reduced sense of smell, and what are some of the likely causes to disrupt the sense of smell?	• Hyposmia (reduced) Anosmia (complete) • Rhinosinusitis with or without polyps • Idiopathic • Pregnancy • Trauma • Neoplasia – intranasal or intracranial • Congential abnormality
Competency question(s)	**Answer**
What other medical terms are you aware of to describe disruption to one's sense of	• Anosmia – no sense. Seen in trauma or congenital abnormalities • Hyposmia – reduced sense. Seen in smokers, increasing age, disease processes

smell?	• Hyperosmia – increased sense. Seen in hunger, pregnancy or endocrine disorders (Addison's disease) • Phantosmia – olfactory hallucinations (intracerebral tumours) • Dysosmia – disordered sense (during neural degeneration/recovery) • Parosmia – change in quality (dementia) • Cacosmia – foul smell Seen in acute or chronic rhinosinisitis, infections
How would you investigate hyposmia?	<u>Smell Tests</u> • **UPSIT** (University of Pennsylvania Smell Identification Test) Uses microencapsulated odours which are released by scratching standardised odour-impregnated test booklets (some smells 'Americanised') • **Sniffin' Sticks** Pen-like odour dispensing devices which are used to assess olfactory threshold, discrimination and identification. • **Combined Olfactory Test** The test consists of an odour recognition test of nine odours (i.e. coffee, engine oil, etc), where an odour in a bottle is chosen from a list of four possible odours in a forced choice manner. This is followed by a threshold test using a series of three-fold dilutions of 1-butanol. The mean of the two scores is the combined olfactory score.

<table>
<tr><td></td><td>

- **Smell Diskettes**

Reusable diskettes as applicators of 8 different odorants (coffee, vanilla, smoke, peach, pineapple, rose, coconut, vinegar). Using a questionnaire with illustrations, the test was designed as a triple forced multiple choice test resulting in a score of 0 to 8

- **Threshold (Doty) Bottles**
- **Olfactometers**

<u>Cross-sectional Radiology</u>

- CT – exclude paranasal sinus disease, trauma
- MRI – intracranial pathology

<u>Blood Tests</u>

- Thyroid Function Tests
- ACE/ANCA
- Zinc

</td></tr>
<tr><th>Advanced question(s)</th><th>Answer</th></tr>
<tr><td>

What is the spherical structure on the septum of this patient?

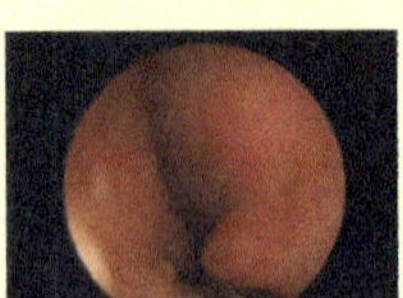

</td><td>

<u>Vomeronasal organ (VNO)</u>

- The vomeronasal (or Jacobson's) organ is an extra olfactory sense organ on the nasal septum found in animals, believed to be involved in the detection of pheromones.
- The receptors contained in this area arise from those found in the olfactory system. The VNO appears as a pit on either side

</td></tr>
</table>

	of the nasal septum. Unlike the olfactory bulb, which sends neuronal signals to the olfactory cortex, the VNO sends neuronal signals to the accessory olfactory bulb and ultimately to the hypothalamus. Although chemical communication does appear to occur in humans, it does not imply that the human VNO is functional, and its role remains controversial.

2.9 SEPTAL PERFORATION and SEPTAL BUTTON

CLINICAL PHOTOGRAPH	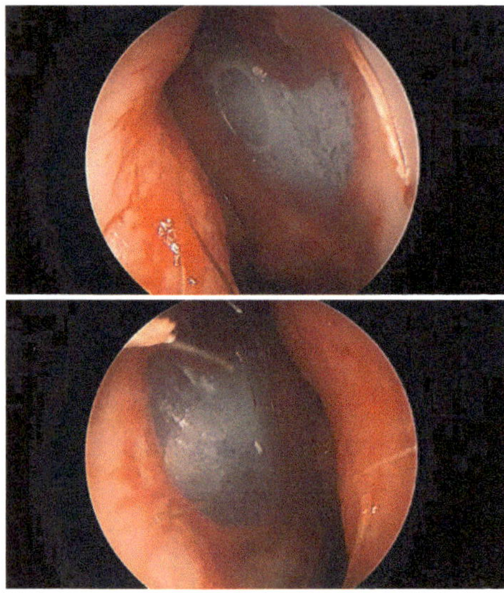

Introductory question	Answer
Describe the photographs	• Right and Left endoscopic views of the septum of the nose showing a septal button *in situ*. • The perforation appears to be quite large, perhaps over 1 cm, which is difficult to correct surgically.

Competency question(s)	Answer
Tell me about the causes for septal perforations.	• **Trauma**: nose picking, septoplasty, nasal cautery, • **Infection:** septal abscess, syphilis, TB • **Chemical irritants**: cocaine, decongestant nasal sprays, chemicals from button batteries. • **Inflammation**: sarcoidosis, Wegener's granulomatosis • **Neoplasia**: SCC adenocarcinoma, melanoma • **Idiopathetic**
How would you attempt to close a small (less than 1cm) septal perforaton	• **Free graft:** simple or composite autografts, allografts, • **Rotation or** advancement of mucoperichondrial or mucoperiosteal flap • **Pedicle flaps:** local nasal mucosa, buccal mucosa, composite septal cartilage
Advanced question(s)	**Answer**
What do you understand by term rhinolalia?	Secondary nasal speech. Rhinolalia clausa is hyponasal speech due to nasal obstruction, eg. polyps, foreign body, adenoid hypertrophy. Rhinolalia aperta is hypernasal speech mainly due to velopharyngeal insufficiency. Large

	perforation of the septum may lead to rhinolalia aperta.

Also available:

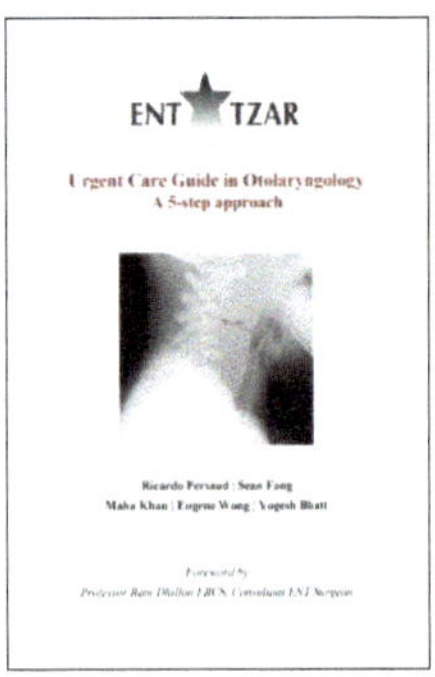

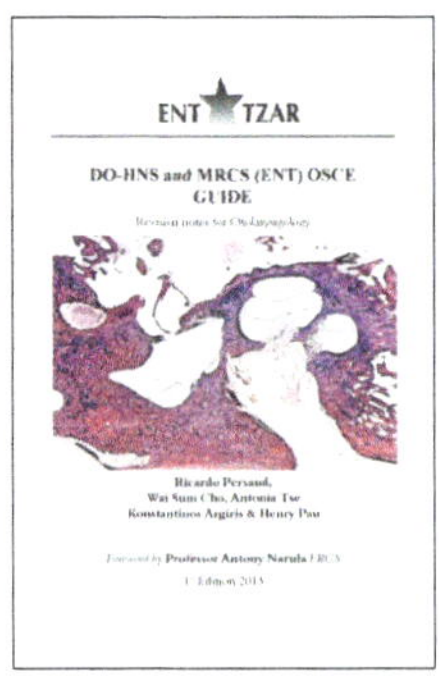

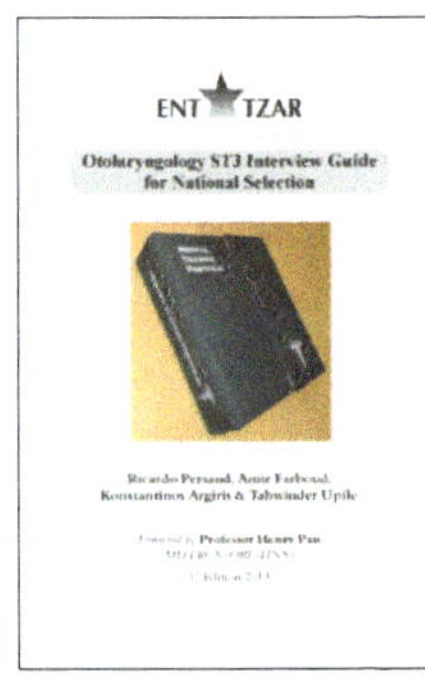

2.10 NASAL TRAUMA

CLINICAL PHOTOGRAPH	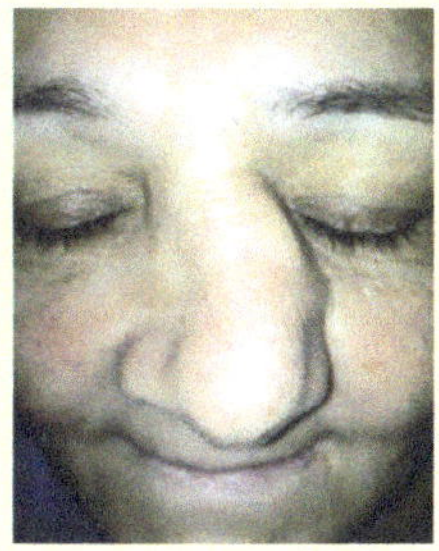

Introductory question	Answer
Describe what you see in the clinical photograph?	• Clinical photograph showing gross C-shape deviation of the nose to the left with significant distortions of the brow tip aesthetic lines on both sides, especially the upper and middle third of the nose. The nasal bones and the upper lateral cartilages are all involved in the deformity.
The above patient was referred for a septorhinoplasty procedure after years of domestic abuse. What is important in the history?	• Premorbid shape of the nose, mechanism of injury, whether physical abuse has been dealt with and situation resolved before surgery.
Competency question(s)	**Answer**

You examine her nose and found a septal perforation in the absence of previous surgery. What may be the cause? How would you ensure that the patient is not using cocaine? What test would the GP request for cocaine?	• This may be due to previous trauma, due to autoimmune disease such as Wegeners, sarcoidosis, infection or secondary to drug abuse. • Ask the patient directly, write to GP, GP needs to carry out tests to ensure she is drug-free for 1 year before reconstructive surgery. • Urine, saliva, blood tests;
Advanced question(s)	**Answer**
What other test can the GP undertake?	• Cocaine can be tested for in hair for up to 90 days.

2.11 LIMITED WEGENER'S DISEASE

SCENARIO **(no clinical photograph)**	You are referred a 50-yr-old man with persistent excessive nasal crusting and epistaxis.

Introductory question	Answer
What is your differential diagnosis?	• Infections • Traumatic perforation • Wegener's granulomatosis (WG) • Sarcoidosis • Atrophic rhinitis • Sino-nasal malignancy
Competency question(s)	**Answer**
How would you manage this patient?	• **History** –nasal surgery, trauma (including digital), topical drugs, symptoms of connective tissue disease (especially respiratory), and symptoms of local spread including visual impairment/diplopia, facial numbness. • **Examination** – 3 pass nasendoscopy, focused cranial nerve examination for

	local extension, CXR and urinalysis for WG and sarcoid. • **Investigations** – nasal biopsy for histology and culture with imaging guided by clinical signs. Serology is essential. cANCA, ANA, Rheumatoid Factor plus serum ACE. CXR and urinalysis obligatory. • **Treatment** – Guided by underlying diagnosis. WG/sarcoidosis managed in conjunction with rheumatologists etc. Basic hygiene with decrusting and nasal douching +/- antibiotics guided by swabs. Septal button as first line management of symptomatic perforation.
Advanced question(s)	**Answer**
The cANCA returns positive. What is the role of antibiotic therapy in managing this patient?	• Wegener's is a systemic autoimmune vasculitic condition affecting the upper and lower airways and causing necrotising glomerulonephritis. • cANCA immunofluorescent pattern is due to antibody reactivity against the leukocyte proteinase-3 protein (PR3). This is also known as Myeloblastin. • Most patients with WG are colonised with Staph. aureus. Evidence suggests that this may promote disease flares. Co-trimoxazole may suppress these. • Sino-nasal 'mucosal failure' manifesting as atrophic rhinitis is associated with Klebsiella ozaenae which may be controlled by quinolone antibiotics.

2.12 SYSTEMIC WEGENER'S GRANULOMATOSIS (GRANULOMATOSIS POLYANGIITIS, GPA)

SCENARIO **(no clinical photograph)**	You are asked to see a patient on the medical ward with renal failure who is having intermittent epistaxis. On examination there is nasal crusting with a friable mucosa.

Introductory question	Answer
What is your differential diagnosis?	• Infections • Traumatic perforation • Wegener's granulomatosis (WG) • Sarcoidosis • Atrophic rhinitis • Sino-nasal malignancy
Competency question(s)	**Answer**
Tell me about Wegner's Granulomatosis?	**Background** • Unknown aetiology – possibly autoimmune • Idiopathic necrotising granulomatous vasculitis • Multinucleated giant cells which may affect upper and lower respiratory tracts

	and may also cause necrotising glomerulonephritis • Affects upper and lower respiratory tracts • Causes glomerulonephritis • Limited – no renal involvement Systemic – renal involvement **Symptoms** • Haemoptysis, cough, dyspnoea • Haematuria • Fever, night sweats • Arthralgia/myalgia • Cutaneous lesions **Signs** • Epistaxis, nasal obstruction, rhinosinusitis, septal ulceration/perforation • Subglottic stenosis • Uveitis • Hearing loss (CHL/SNHL) **Investigations** • cANCA and PR3 (86% specific) • Biopsy (lung – highest yield, renal – if glomerulonephritis, nasal – poor yield) **Prognosis very poor if left untreated**

Advanced question(s)	Answer
What are the diagnostic options here, when would you perform a nasal septal biopsy, and what are the treatment options for this condition?	If diagnosis equivocal despite cANCA/PR3 and the nasal septal mucosa appearance shows hypererythema or irregularity, then a nasal septal biopsy could be performed. This often gives a poor diagnostic yield as it is often obscured by inflammatory cells. Pulmonary or renal biopsy are other possibilities but carry higher morbidity. Treatment can be in the form of administering: • Steroids • Cyclophosphamide • Azathioprine • Methotrexate

2.13 EMPTY NOSE SYNDROME

SCENARIO	A 47-year old man has been referred back to your clinic 2 years after having had sinonasal surgery for nasal obstruction. He complains bitterly of nasal congestion, scabbing and dryness. 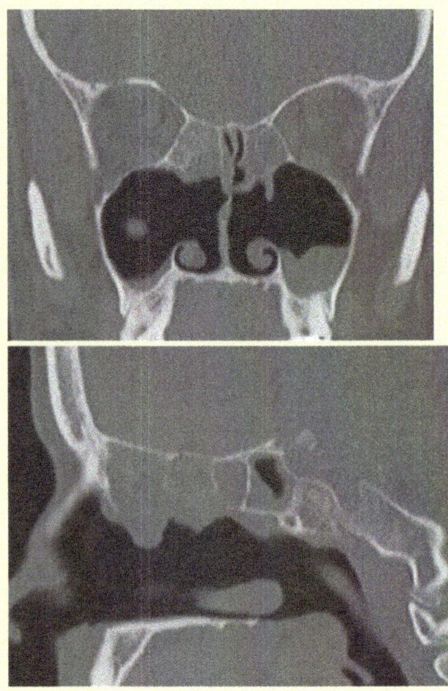

Introductory question	**Answer**
Describe what	• Coronal and sagital sections showing loss of mucosal surfaces necessary to

you see?	humidify inhaled air • This may result in empty nose syndrome and atrophic rhinitis
Competency question(s)	**Answer**
What is empty nose syndrome? How would you manage this patient?	• It is a recognised complication of sinonasal surgery, especially following radical turbinectomy. The absence of normal nasal structures is universal in these patients, and the symptoms of atrophic rhinitis coupled with a cavernous nasal airway lacking identifiable turbinate tissue has been termed the empty nose syndrome. • Managing this condition is challenging and the evidence base for most treatment modalities remains low. • Recommended conservative management does not differ significantly from atrophic rhinitis and includes a combination nasal lavage, lubricant drops and topical corticosteroids. • Surgical intervention for ENS aims to increase nasal airway resistance by narrowing the nasal valve region or to reconstruct the resected turbinate.
Advanced question(s)	**Answer**

How would you manage hypertrophy of the inferior turbinate?	• Conservative: topical steroids. • Surgery: Numerous techniques, mostly technology driven, such as laser, Coblation, turbinoplasty have been described. However, few studies have evaluated clinical outcomes using objective measures of nasal airflow such as rhinomanometry. The randomised clinical study undertaken by Passàli D et al. (2003) reported that submucosal resection and outfracture of the inferior turbinate resulted in optimal long-term normalization of nasal patency and in restoration of mucociliary clearance at up to 6 years follow-up.

2.14 FRONTAL MUCOCOELE

SCENARIO **(followed by a clinical photograph)**	This 58-year old woman was referred from the ophthalmologist with gradually progressing diplopia, proptosis and a swelling over his left eye.

Introductory question	**Answer**
How would you assess this patient?	• Full history focusing on her current sinonasal symptoms and visual problems, previous history of craniofacial trauma, sinonasal surgery, sinus pathology (e.g. nasal polyposis, Samster's, systemic vasculitis), smoking, occupation (e.g. hard wood worker, exposure to toxic fumes). • Full ENT examination including endoscopy of the nasal cavities.
Competency question(s)	**Answer**
This patient gives a 6 months history of nasal congestion and headache. She had endoscopic sinus surgery	• Coronal CT scan showing a smooth, homogenous lesion in the left frontal sinus, extending into the left orbit. There is bony erosion over the supraorbital rim. The globe appears to be displaced downwards compared to the opposite side. There is a rim of thin bone at the

several years ago for chronic rhinosinusitis with polyps, and had been on topical treatment since. Describe what you see in this scan. 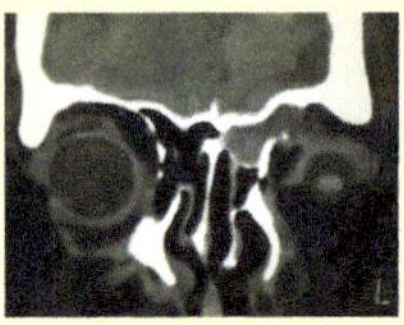 What do you think has happened to this patient? How would you manage this patient?	bottom of the lesion. There is evidence of previous sinus surgery as the anterior ethmoid cells have been excised. • This is likely a frontal mucocele, secondary to scarring/ stenosis of the frontal sinus outflow tract. Pressure effect of the mucocele causes bony erosion and remodelling. There may even be reversible palsy of the trochlear nerve supplying superior oblique muscle, resulting in diplopia and difficulty walking down stairs. • She will require surgery to drain the mucocele. This can be undertaken as an external approach (e.g. Lynch-Howarth incision) or endoscopically (e.g. Draf IIb, III). Prophylactic antibiotics remains contentious and should be withheld if the patient is asymptomatic Consider referring the patient to a rhinologist. A MRI scan may be required to determine the entent of the mucocele and there should be discussion with the ophthalmologist to discuss reconstruction of the defect on the outer table, if necessary

Advanced question(s)	Answer
What would you do if whilst waiting for surgery, she presents with acute swelling, headache, pyrexia and photophobia?	• I would be concerned that the mucocele may become infected i.e mucopyocele. • This patient requires admission, intravenous antibiotics and urgent scans (CT and MRI). Depending on the radiological findings, I may be to confer with my ophthalmologist and neurosurgical colleagues. Nevertheless, this patient would require emergent surgery in the form of external drainage (via a Lynch-Howarth incision). • An endoscopic approach to re-establish intra-nasal drainiage should be considered, or seek help from a more experienced colleague after the acute infection has been drained.

2.15 INVERTED PAPILLOMA

SCENARIO FOLLOWED BY A CLINICAL PHOTOGRAPH	A 45 year old man is referred from his GP. In the clinic letter, the GP has diagnosed a "unilateral nasal polyp" in the left nasal cavity and asks for further management. The patient has been suffering with unilateral nasal obstruction, cacosmia and occasional epistaxis.

Introductory question	Answer
What is your differential diagnosis?	• Benign: Simple inflammatory polyps (e.g large antrochoanal polyp), inverted papilloma, angiofibroma, granulomatous lesion, tuberculous • Malignant (primary or secondary): squamous cell carcinoma, adenocarcinoma, met from kidney or elsewhere in the body)
How would you assess this patient?	• The history should concentrate on sinonasal symptoms: rhinorhoea, obstruction, pain, pressure, epistaxis, reduction in sense of smell, excessive itching and sneezing. Visual disturbance and previous sinus

	surgery as well as significant past medical history are also relevant. • Full ENT Examination including endoscopy of the nasal and nasopharyngeal regions.
Competency question(s)	**Answer**
Describe what you see. 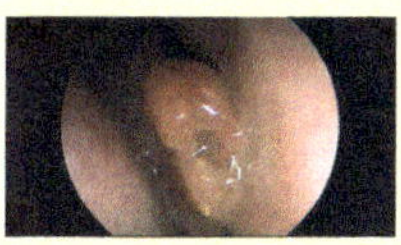 How would you investigate this patient? Why MRI scan? Biopsies have confirmed inverted papilloma and imaging shows no invasion of the orbit or skull base. Where is the most common site of	• This is an endoscopic view of the right nasal cavity; the septum is on the right and the middle turbinate is on the left. • There is a fleshy/polypoidal mass originating from the lateral wall, blocking the middle meatus. It does not appear to be vascular and the surface appears to be lined with squamous epithelium. • At this stage, my working diagnosis is either inverted papilloma or a malignant sinonasal tumour and therefore I would request a CT and MRI of the nose and paranasal sinus and then a biopsy of the lesion under a general anaesthesia in theatre, if I am convinced it is not a juvenile angiofibroma. • It is good for defining soft tissue lesion and inverted papilloma has a characteristic cerebriform (brain-like)

origin for inverted papilloma? How would you manage this patient?	appearance. • Lateral nasal wall, followed by maxillary and ethmoid sinuses. True frontal sinus inverted papilloma is uncommon. • Endoscopic surgical resection is appropriate for most lesions (e.g medial maxillectomy, full-house FESS, Draf III), external approach (e.g lateral rhinotomy, craniofacial resection for frontal sinus disease or extensive skull base involvement). A Caldwell - Luc and/or septotomy could also be undertaken to improve exposure to facilitate resection. The site of origin may be identified on CT scans (an area suggestive of osteitis) and should be drilled to prevent recurrence. • Follow-up: You would recommend long-term review for recurrence. The European position paper suggest 3 years follow-up.
Advanced question(s)	**Answer**
What classification system do you know for inverted	• Krause system • Yes, the literature states that the incidence of synchronous and metachronous carcinoma to be approximately 5-10 percent.

papilloma? Is there malignant potential with inverted papilloma? What is the role of radiotherapy in treating inverted papilloma?	However, it should be remembered that this data is based in a review of tertiary departments and the incidence could be biased. • The evidence for using radiotherapy in the primary treatment of inverted papilloma. The issue of radiotherapy in extensive disease following surgical resection remains contentious. This decision is predicated on the severity of metaplasia and dysplasia in the histological samples, and should be duly discussed in a multidisciplinary setting.

2.16 ATROPHIC RHINITIS

SCENARIO	A 45 year old man from the middle east presents with nasal obstruction epistaxis, anosmia, foul smelling green, yellow crusts and occasional choking episodes. He previously had FESS, reduction of concha bullosa and resection of his inferior turbinates.

Introductory question	Answer
What is going through your mind with the above history? Why is he having choking episodes?	• Atrophic rhinitis would be my main concern • I would also be thinking of granulomatous diseases such as Wegeners, sarcoidosis, syphilis, leprosy and TB. • Crust from the nose obstructing the larynx

Competency question(s)	Answer
What is the cause of atrophic rhinitis? Tell me about treatment of atrophic rhinitis.	• Primary cases may arise denovo and is common in India and Middle East. Role of coccobacillus and Klebsiella unclear but these organisms are frequently present in atrophic rhinitis • Secondary cases are seen in developed countries and may be iatrogenic – due to excessive destruction of turbinates by surgery or after irradiation therapy. • Nasal douche, antibiotics, vitamin A, glucose in glycerine • Submucous injections of paraffin • teflon strips, and autogenous cartilages grafting • Submucosal injection of 50% Teflon in glycerin paste • Repeated stellate ganglion blocks (causes imbalance in favour of parasympathetic activity in nose) • Young's operation (reopen 6-9 months) (Nb many believe steroids to be contraindicated)

Advanced question(s)	Answer
What are the CT findings in	• Thickening of sinuses

atrophic rhinitis?	• Resorption of bulla and uncinate • poorly defined OMC • Hypoplastic maxilla • Erosion of lat nasal wall and atrophy of turbinates.

2.17 CAVERNOUS SINUS THROMBOSIS

SCENARIO FOLLOWED BY A CLINICAL PHOTOGRAPH	A 23 year old university student presents with progressively increasing sharp headache in the regions of the eyes and upper face over the last 48 hours. She suffers with severe acne and recently developed a furuncle on the cheek. She denies any symptoms of rhinosinusitis. Rhinological and dental examinations were completely normal but examination of the eyes reveals evidence of bilateral chemosis.

Introductory question	**Answer**
What do you think is the cause for her symptoms?	• The history is typical of someone with potential cavernous sinus thrombosis.
Competency question(s)	**Answer**
Which organism is most commonly associated with cavernous sinus thrombosis? Apart from the	• 70% Staph aureus is responsible for up to 70% of cavernous sinus thrombosis, other organisms include s.pneumoniae, anaerobes and fungi. • sinuses (sphenoid, ethmoid, or frontal) • dental abscess, nares, tonsils, soft palate,

face, which other regions be the source of infections? What is the mechanism for the chemosis? If left untreated what other symptoms might she develop?	middle ear, or orbit (orbital cellulitis) • obstruction of the ophthalmic veins • sixth nerve palsy leading to double vision • 3rd nerve palsy leading to ptosis, mydriasis, alterned eye movements • Raised IOP (exopthalmos, ophthalmoplegia, sluggish pupils, decreased acuity) • Hypoaesthesia of V1 and V2 • Meningeal and septic signs
Advanced question(s)	**Answer**
Which radiological investigation would you request? What is the treatment?	• CT with contrast as well as MR (MRV) to check for flow voids • High dose broad spectrum antibiotics such as ceftrixone (3-4/52), steroid and heparin.

2.18 POTT'S PUFFY TUMOUR

SCENARIO FOLLOWED BY A CLINICAL PHOTOGRAPH	GP Referral: Dear Dr, Please could you see this gentleman with a forehead lump which appears to be increasing in size over the last 48 hours. The lump is associated with a swinging pyrexia and nasal discharge. He has a history of rhinosinusitis. 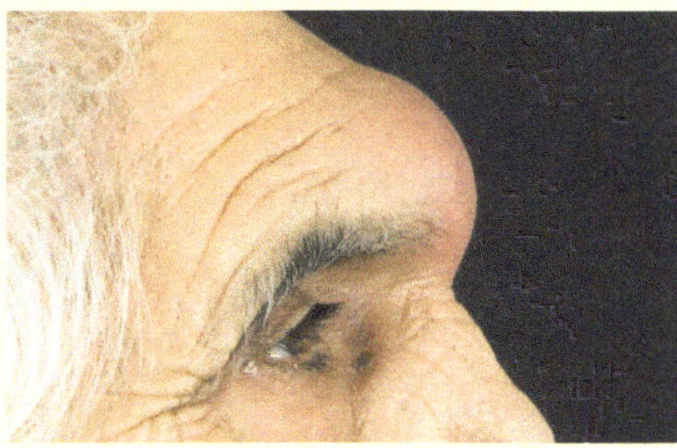

Introductory question	Answer
Based on the history given and the appearance of the lump, what is your differential	• I would be considering an infective or neoplastic process. • For example, frontal sinusitis, Pott's puffy tumour, benign sinus tumour such as a polyp, primary malignancy or

diagnosis?	metastatic disease.
Competency question(s)	**Answer**
How would you reach a diagnosis?	• After taking a full history and performing a full ENT examination I would request: blood profile such as FBC, CRP, ESR and blood culture. • I would take a nasal swab for MC+S • I would also request a contrast CT head and para-nasal sinuses and MRI with contrast brain.
What is Pott's Puffy tumour?	• Pott's Puffy tumour is a subperiosteal collection of pus and an osteomyelitic anterior table of the frontal sinus. • This condition is associated with intracranial complications in 30% of cases and demands an MR brain with contrast enhancement and repeat assessment as symptoms dictate.
How is the condition treated?	• Intracranial complication is indicated by focal neurological symptoms/reduced GCS/raised intracranial pressure. • Prolonged course of IV antibiotics typically for 6 weeks followed by oral step down. • Surgical drainage of pus [via external incision and/or functional endoscopic sinus surgery (FESS)]. • Direct incision may lead to fistulation and

	frontal sinus surgery may be hazardous. • Frontal sinus trephine may represent an effective compromise. • Bony sequestra occasionally require open debridement. • When there are co-existing intracranial complications (30% of cases) treatment is best decided by a multi-professional team involving surgeons, radiologist and microbiologist.
Advanced question(s)	**Answer**
What is the typical microbiological organisms associated with Pott's Puffy tumour?	• Polymicrobial organisms: strep, bacteroides and staphylococci • If intracranial complications are present then the more likely organisms are fusobacter and bacteroides

2.19 ALLERGIC RHINITIS

CLINICAL PHOTOGRAPH	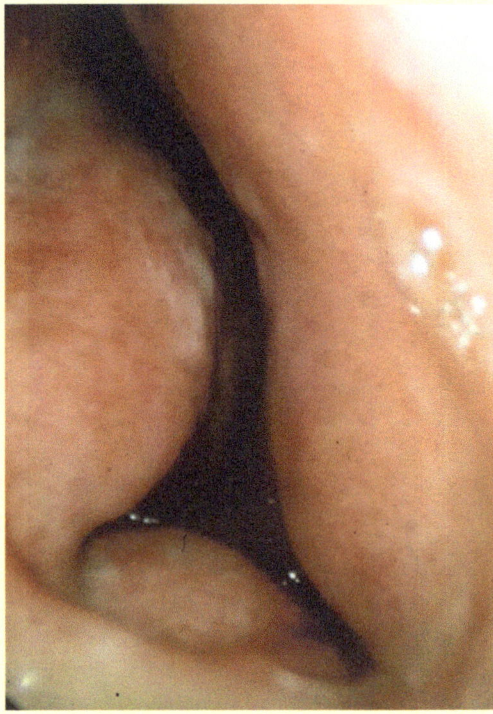

Introductory question	Answer
Describe what you see in the	• Clinical photograph of the right nostril showing enlarged inferior turbinate and

photograph	watery rhinorrhoea • This may represent rhinitis (allergic or infective) or CSF rhinorrhoea
Competency question(s)	**Answer**
How would you attempt to differentiate?	• I would take a full history and perform a full ENT examination • In the history I would like to know about the nature of symptoms colour of d/c, ocular or respiratory symptoms); increase on bending forward, timing (seasons/perennial, outdoor/school/home, exacerbation/alleviation); Duration, FH, Related history (asthma, eczema); Social history (pillows, pets etc.) • On examination I would look for Allergic shiners, Morgan Dennie lines, Allergic salute; Conjuctival erythema; OME, Pale blue enlarged inferior turbinates, Rhinorrhoea, dried blood); high arched palate & discoloured palate = mouth breather; **cobblestoning of posterior pharyngeal wall = PND)** • Skin Prick Test or RAST (or beta 2 transferin if I am concerned about CSF rhinirrhoea)

Advanced question(s)	Answer
What is the immunopathology of allergic rhinitis?	• **Type 1 hypersensitivity reaction**: IgE binds allergen – cross linking causes mast cell degranulation (Fc bound to mast cell) Release of mediators – histamine, prostaglandin D2, tryptase, heparin, PAF, leukotrienes.
What is the treatment recommended by ARIA?	**Stepwise treatment** All patients allergen avoidance based on SPT or RAST • *Mild intermittent* Oral H1 blocker, intranasal H1 blocker, consider decongestant • *Mod/severe intermittent & mild persistent* As above + Intranasal Corticosteroid (CS), if no improvement 4/52 step up • *Mod/severe persistent* Intranasal CS. If no improvement 4/52 (increase IN CS dose, add H1 blocker for itch/sneeze, oral CS, ipratropium for rhinorrhoea) ***Pharmacology:*** Neoclarityn has additional effect on nasal blockage Metanalaysis: Corticosteroid is better than H1 antagonists Beclomethasone has effects on growth Mometasone/fluticasone low bioavailability

	Leucotrienes antagonists + H1 blocker not as good as intranasal corticosteroids.

Also available:

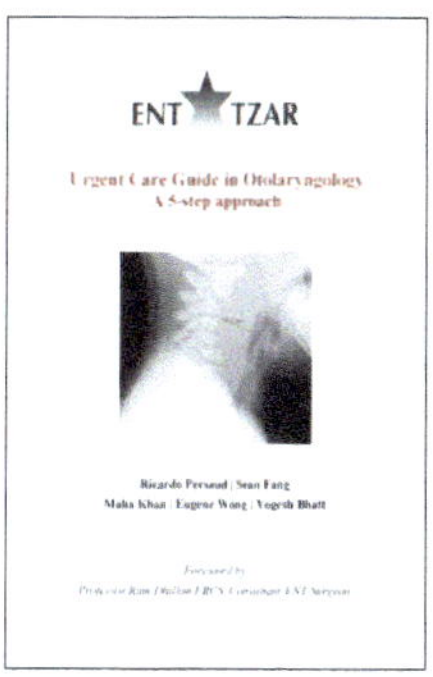

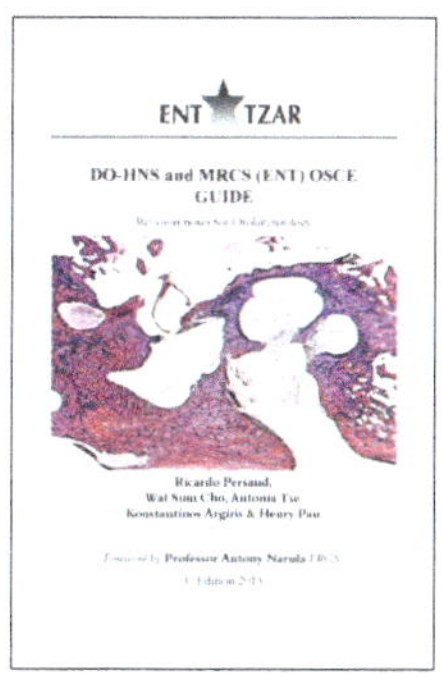

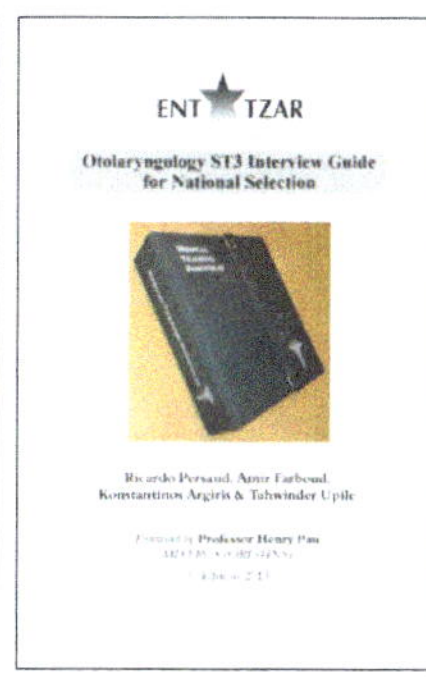

2.20 RHINITIS MEDICAMENTOSA

CLINICAL PHOTOGRAPH	
	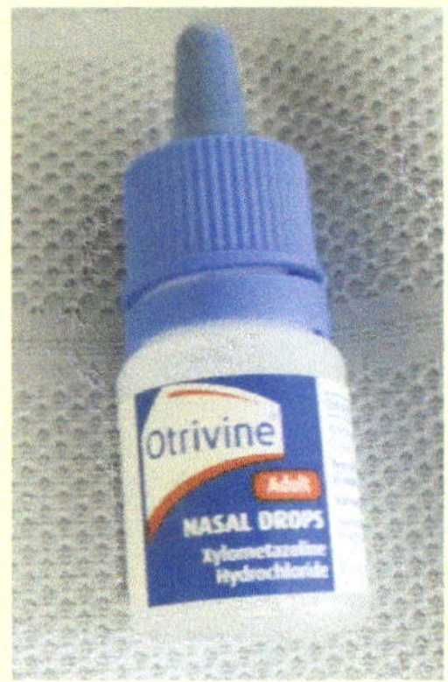

Introductory question	Answer
What is the problem associated with long term usage of the nasal drops shown in the photo?	• The patient will develop rhinitis medicamentosa
Competency question(s)	**Answer**

Tell me more about that condition.	• It is essentially rebound nasal congestion secondary to vasodilatation after topical sympatheticomimetic treatment This may be due to a number of factors: • longer beta effect than alpha effect • prolonged vasoconstriction causes tissue hypoxia and thus reactive hyperaemia • alpha 2 agonists stimulate negative feedback loop at presynaptic terminals • alters vasomotor tone and increase parasympathetic activity
How is the condition treated?	• Patient education • Stop topical decongestants • Sedating anti-histamine at night to help sleep • Nasal douching • Topical nasal corticosteroid • Systemic decongestants in first 1-2 weeks or a short course of oral steroids or im corticosteroid injection eg Deprofos.

Advanced question(s)	Answer
What is the nasal cycle?	• This cycle refers to the turbinate and other nasal mucosa undergoes regular periodic side-to-side or alternate engorgement with blood (note that the turbinates are made of erectile tissue, which also explains honey moon rhinitis). • Cyclical alternate variation of blood flow in the turbinates is present in approximately 80% of people. • Frequency of cycling is 30mins to 5 hours and is specific for an individual • Most active in adolescence and under hypothalamic control • The nasal cycle is linked to the ultradian rhythm of alternating cerebral hemispheric activity. • The sympathetic system regulates blood flow to the nasal mucosa by regulating *resistance* vessels. Increased resistance and thus less flow into the nasal mucosa, leading to decongestion. • The parasympathetic system regulates blood volume of the nasal mucosa by regulating *capacitance* vessels. Leads to relaxation of capacitance vessels, allowing congestion and even edema formation in tissues.

2.21 DISORDER OF SCARRING

CLINICAL PHOTOGRAPH	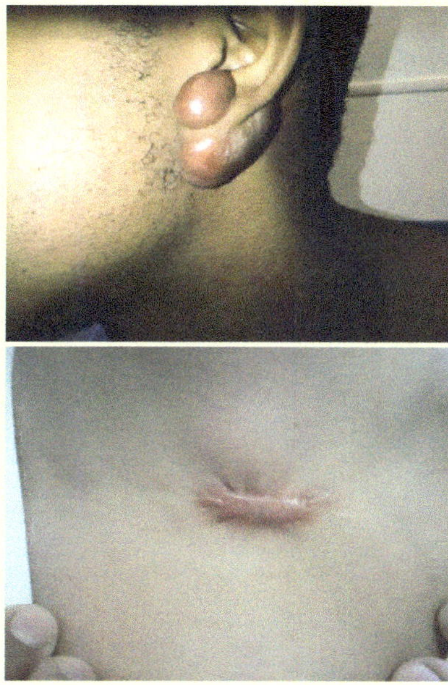

Introductory question	Answer
Describe what you see in the photographs	• A keloid scar because the scar tissue extends beyond the incision • A hypertrohic scar because the scar tissue is confined to the site of the

	incision
Competency question(s)	**Answer**
What is Keloid? Who tends to get keloid? Tell me about the treatment for keloid?	• Keloids are the result of an overgrowth of dense fibrous tissue • Usually develops after healing of a skin injury • Does not usually regress spontaneously • Tends to recur after excision • Variation in normal healing. At 6-8weeks catabolic and anabolic processes in equilibrium. If more anabolic (ie more collagen deposition) will lead to disorder of scarring (hypertrophic/keloid scar). • 16% of Blacks. Highest incidence 10-20yrs. F>M (due to earlobe piercing) • Prevention is better than cure so if possible avoid surgery, unnecessary piercing etc, apply minimal tension in sutures during surgery and try not cross joints (contractures) In general, large unsightly keloid is managed by surgical excision and one of the following: • Compression/occlusive dressings • Triamcinolone 10-40mg every 6/52 • Silicone gel • Interferon • Radiotherapy

Advanced question(s)	Answer
Any other treatment available?	• Verapamil (Blocks synthesis and secretion of extracellular matrix molecules) • Bleomycin (Injections cause necrosis of keratinocytes) • 5FU (inhibits fibroblastic proliferation) • Retinoic acid derivatives, immune modulators

2.22 SEPTORHINOPLASTY

CLINICAL PHOTOGRAPHS	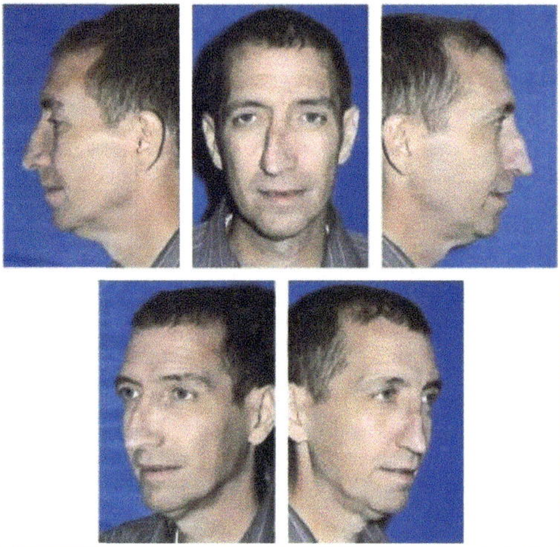

Introductory question	Answer
Talk me through the assessment of the nose for septorhinoplasty with reference to the patient seen in the	This patient appear to have a left sided deviated nasal pyramid with a dorsal hump; the nose also appear to be long although the nasolabial angle is about 90 degrees. I would assess further in terms of: **Horizontal Thirds** • Upper – trichion to glabella

photographs. Tell me about the lines and angles relevant to septorhinoplasty	• Middle – glabella to sub-nasale • Lower – sub-nasale to menton **Vertical Fifths** • Width of nose = width of eyes = width of lateral canthus to ear **Lines and angles** • Frankfort horizontal line = Superior point of auditory canal to most inferior point of infra-orbital rim; this is important for clinical photograph before and after surgery • Facial line is a vertical line from the glabella perpendicular through Frankfort horizontal and ideally should touch the anterior chin; hence indicating if there is excessive protrusion or retraction of the chin. • Nasofrontal Angle = 115-130 degrees (angle defined by glabella-nasion line intersecting nasion-tip line) • Nasofacial Angle = 30-40 degrees (angle defined by glabella-pagonion line intersecting tip-pagonion line) • Nasomental Angle =120-132 degrees (angle defined by nasion-tip line intersecting tip-pagonion line) • Nasolabial Angle = 90-110 degrees (95-110 for females) • Columullar show 2-4mm on profile view

	• Nasal Projection - Goode's Method: ratio of (nasal tip to alar line) to (nasion to nasal tip line); normal is 0.55-0.60
Competency question(s)	**Answer**
How would correct the deformities mentioned?	• Open approach via inverted V and marginal incisions • Nasal laparotomy • Isolate the septal cartilage (and perform septoplasty if necessary) • Division of upper lateral cartilages (ULCs) from septum bilaterally • The cartilage of the hump is incised with a scalpel; this creates a joint at the junction of the bone and cartilage • An osteotome is used on the bony dorsal hump • The bone cartilage hump is removed in one piece. • Rasp if necessary • Trim upper lateral cartilage as required • Medial and lateral osteotomies to close open roof deformity • Secure ULC to septum with or without spreader grafts

Advanced question(s)	Answer
What are the advantages and disadvantages of the endonasal (closed) vs open septorhinoplasty?	**Advantages of endonasal (closed) approach** • less dissection • less swelling • less internal and external scarring or flap necrosis • more immediate and predictable ability to feel changes made • shorter operating time • decreased morbidity • quicker return to normal appearance • no post-operative nasal tip numbness **Advantages of open approach** • direct exposure, inspection and assessment of nasal framework • precise modification and stabilisation of the abnormality • better results if patient for thick nasal skill • can deal with difficult nasal tip, eg shield graft option • easier to insert and secure spreader grafts • can address internal nasal valve dysfunction

	• revision surgery • good tool for training

2.23 SADDLE NOSE DEFORMITY

CLINICAL PHOTOGRAPHS	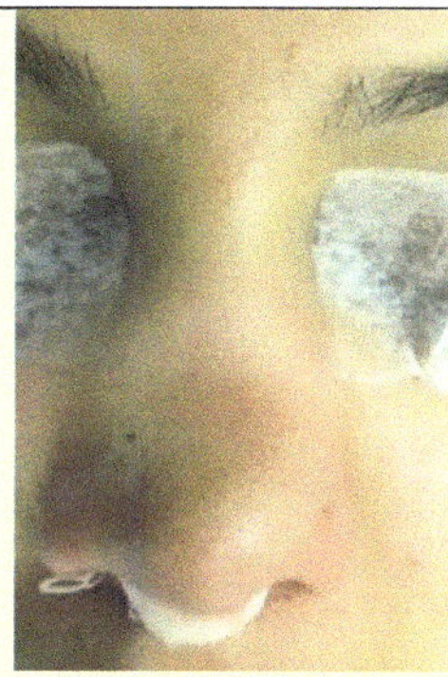 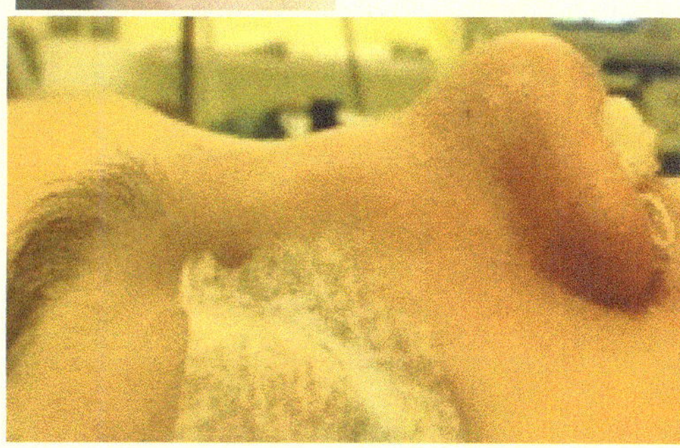

Introductory question	Answer
Describe the abnormality present in the	• Saddle nose deformity

photographs	
Competency question(s)	**Answer**
What are the caused for this deformity How would you investigate this patient? What operation would you do to correct the deformity	The causes may be surgical or medical • Rhinoplasty or SMR (0.4%) • Wegeners – necrotising granulomas and vasculitis of upper and lower respiratory tracts. • Relapsing polychondritis – recurrent episodes of AI catrilage inflammation and destruction, • Substance abuse such a s cocaine • Syphilis – intranasal ulcerative lesions that lead to osteo-chondritis • Leprosy • Ectodermal dysplasia • Photographs, C-ANCA, autoimmune screen, VDRL, leprosy serology • Augmentation septorhinoplasty

Advanced question(s)	Answer
What would be contraindications for surgical correction?	• Chronic autoimmune disease • ongoing cocaine usage • poor peri-operative risk • relative = multiple previous rhinoplasties and boxers)

2.24 NASAL RECONSTRUCTION AFTER TRAUMA

CLINICAL PHOTOGRAPH	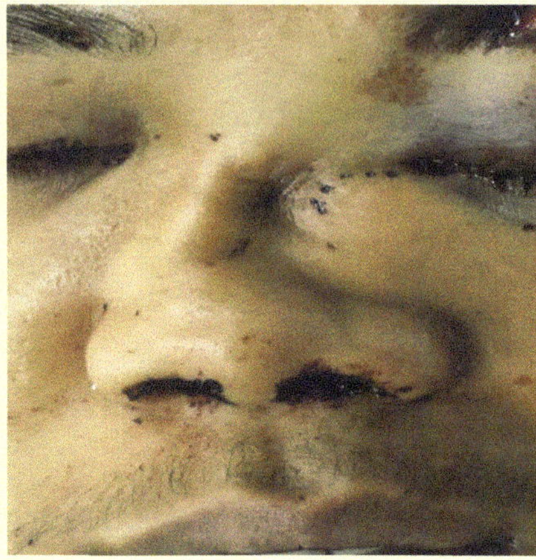

Introductory question	Answer
This man has been referred to you following a drug-related assault. Describe what you see in this picture.	• Grossly deviated nose to the right. • Depressed nasal bone on the left. • Bilateral distortion of the brow-tip aesthetic lines • Soft tissue bruising, lacerations etc.

Competency question(s)	Answer
How would you manage this patient?	• **History** – focusing on the trauma event, clear rhinorrhoea (CSF, skull base fracture), visual problems e.g. diplopia (blow out fracture), sinonasal symptoms (septal hematoma, perforation), • **Examination** – septum, skin over nasal dorsum (thick, sebaceous, mobile, scars), alar cartilages (keystone area), nasal tip. • **Clinical photographs** - remember to obtain consent. Standard views from the front, profile, oblique, basilar and from the top. • Empathetic discussion of issues which concern the patient (aesthetics, functional) and realistic expectations of nasal surgery. • Given that this was an assault, enquire about psychological needs and refer if necessary • It may be necessary to have any psychological assessments complete before proceeding with surgery. There may be need to apply for commissioners for funding; so explain that surgery should not be rushed. Furthermore, the nasal reconstruction required by this patient is complex and will require time to plan or even refer on to a more experienced facial plastics colleague.

Advanced question(s)	Answer
How would you surgically manage this patient?	• Given the complexity of the nasal deformity, an external approach would be more appropriate. This would give opportunity to deal with the septum, bony pyramid and also the nasal tip. • Autologous cartilage grafts can be obtained from the nasal septum, pinna or even costochondral rib. • The nasal tip may require a spreader graft to open up the nasal valve region, or may require inter/intra-domal sutures to improve definition of the bulbous tip, or may require more support with a strut graft. • Shield grafts can be used to smooth out depressions of the nasal dorsum. • Osteotomies will be required to reset the bony pyramid.

2.25 ALAR BASAL CELL CARCINOMA

CLINICAL PHOTOGRAPH	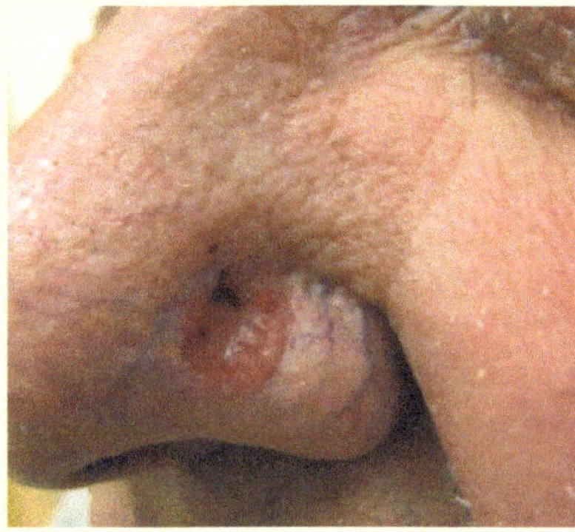

Introductory question	Answer
A 55 year old man has noticed an area of ulceration on the side of his nose. Describe the clinical photograph.	• Lateral/oblique view of patient with lesion on left alar side wall. Well circumscribed, ulcerated centre. • Comment also on any other relevant abnormal features or pathology seen as at this stage you do not consider MOHs first for complete excision. Know what it is that the examiner wants to ask you about, hence cover your bases. Focus in however on the most obvious abnormality.

Competency question(s)	Answer
What is the differential diagnosis? How would you reach a diagnosis? Assuming biopsy confirms a BCC with a morpheaform component, what would your treatment be? What are your reconstructive options in this area?	• **Differential**: infective (eg. TB), traumatic, neoplastic (BCC, SCC, amelanotic melanoma) • **Diagnosis:** The discussion is between an incision vs excision biopsy. Given this is a complex reconstructive area, incision biopsy may be preferable so that definitive therapy can be planned once histology is known. Alar rim lesion / BCC • **Treatment** partly depends on the extent and depth of the lesion. It will need to be excised, then the defect reconstructed. This will in turn depend on the depth of the lesion as a multiple layer reconstruction may be required, with each layer having several options available. • **Reconstruction** - Discuss reconstructive ladder for outer (skin) layer – secondary intention (not good here due to size and location), primary closure (not possible), grafting (SSG or FTSG), local flap (discuss options further – bilobed or nasolabial), distant flap (not necessary). - Inner lining: usually septal mucosa is used, although an inner lining can also be created by fashioning a flap immediately adjacent to, and similar in size as, the excised segment (ideally within the same

	subunit) and inverting it such that the outer skin becomes the inner lining of the defect. This effectively doubles the size of the outer (lateral) defect which can then be reconstructed as above. - Middle layer: usually cartilage either from septum or ear. • Alternatively a **composite graft** such as from the pinna can be used for two of the layers. Also, if the middle and inner linings have been taken care of, a forehead flap can be used if the skin defect is larger than can be accommodated by a local nasal or facial flap.
Advanced question(s)	**Answer**
What about if it was an SCC?	• Skin MDT • Offer RXT to avoid complex reconstruction.

2.26 PINNAPLASTY

SCENARIO **(and clinical photographs)**	GP referral: Many thanks for seeing this 8 year old boy who has prominent ears and whose parents are seeking advice regarding surgical correction. 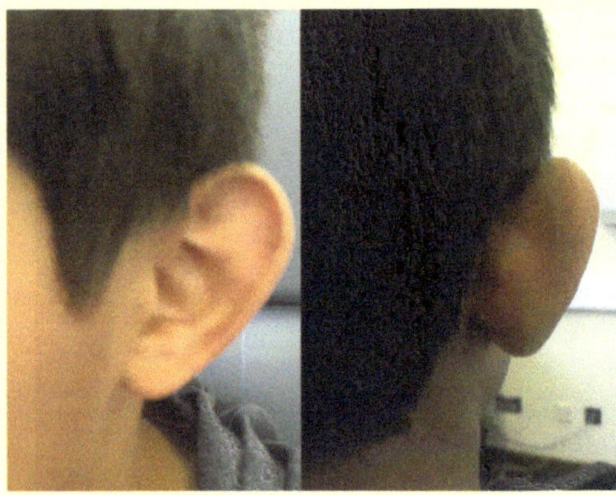

Introductory question	Answer
Described what you see in the photographs.	• Clinical photographs of a young man showing prominent pinnae with underdevelopment of antihelical fold and overdeveloped conchal bowls. Lobules are normal. • Although a lateral view of the ear may appear normal, it is likely that the concha-scaphoid angle will be greater

	than 90 degrees and this suggests a protruding ear.
Competency question(s)	**Answer**
What methods of correction do you know?	• At birth – banding can be attempted but success is dependent on early intervention. • Malleable splints, such as Ear Buddies™ can be taped to the pinna to refashion the antihelical fold. These are usually applied for 2 weeks and can be repeated as necessary. With persistence, splintage can still be effective up to the age of two years, but the process is much more difficult as the infant is by then able to reach up to the ears and potentially interfere with the splints. • Later in childhood – **Surgery:** There are numerous techniques and modifications in current practice to correct prominent ears. Nevertheless, these fall into either Mustade or Scoring.
What are the complications of pinnaplasty?	**Mustarde** technique (posteriorly placed sutures to create the antihelical fold) Anterior cartilage scoring (described by **Chongchet**, Stenstrom) technique.
What else is important to consider pre-operatively?	• These procedures can be carried out under local anaesthetic, but in young children a general anaesthetic is usually required. Other methods to weaken cartilage can be employed (eg. Drilling).

	• Complications – bleeding/infection/scar, telephone ear, over or under-correction, late failure, hypertrophic/keloid scar, tattooing of skin, extrusion of suture material. • Explore concerns of the child and parents e.g. bullying.self awareness.
Advanced question(s)	**Answer**
What do you do about a prominent conchal bowl and lobular protrusion?	• Prominent conchal bowl: 1. Furnas conchomastoid suture – the success of this depends on being able to site the mastoid end of the suture as posteriorly as possible. Also a deep bite of the mastoid periostium is important for good anchorage; 2. Conchal reduction: this is often required along with a Furnas suture for hypertrophy of the conchal bowl as Furnas suturing alone will not always correct this. • Lobular protrusion 1. lobulomastoid setback suture (analogous to the Furnas suture described above); 2. excision of the cauda helicis (the most inferiorly situated piece of conchal cartilage just superior to the soft lobule).

2.27 RHOMBOID FLAP

SCENARIO (and surgical photographs)	Following discussion at the skin MDT meeting, surgery was recommended for the BCC lesion on the right temple of this patient. 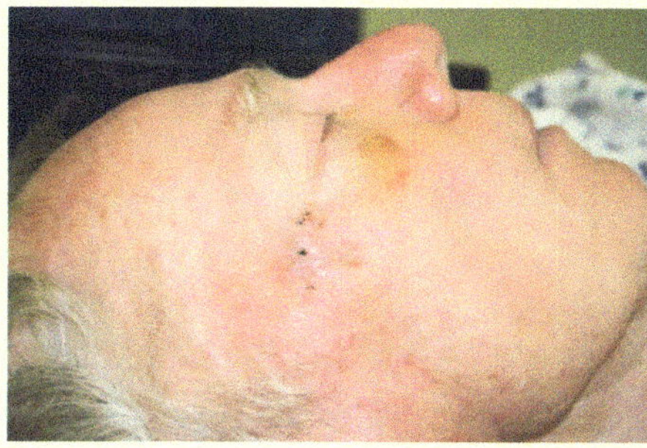

Introductory question	**Answer**
How would you excise the lesion and reconstruct the defect?	• Generally, excised lesions on the temple are best reconstructed using a rhomboid transposition flap. • This involves excising the lesion in a rhomboid shape with 60 and 120 degree angles and then using one of the 4 options with the least tension and cosmetic disruption.

Competency question(s)	Answer
Please draw me how you would perform the excision and use a rhomboid flap.	• The following drawings need to be converted to line diagrams 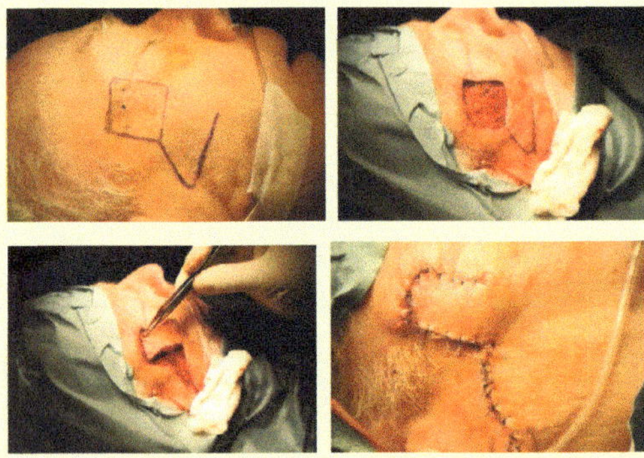 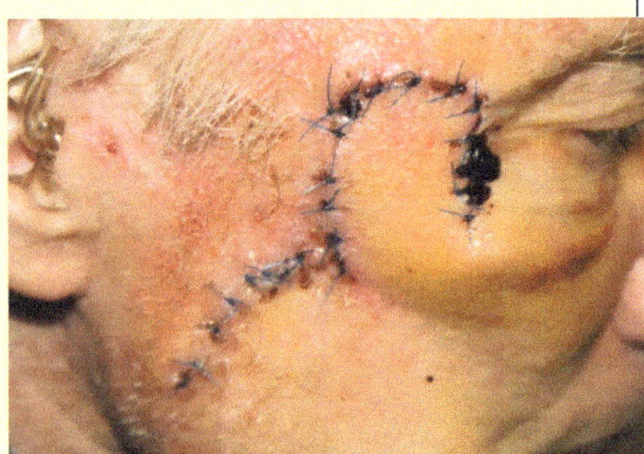

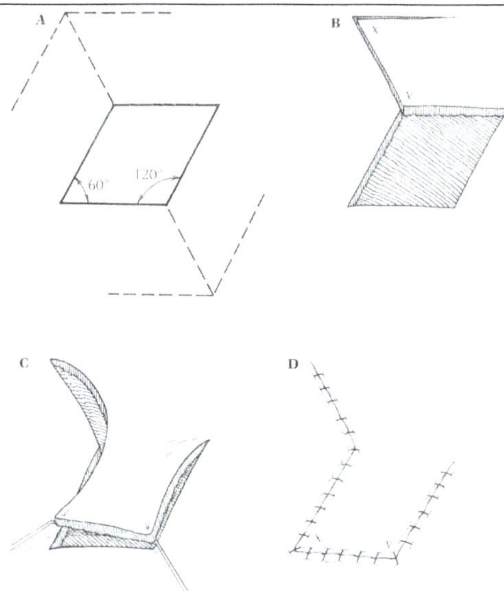

An easy way to remember how to draw it quickly is illustrated in the diagram below.

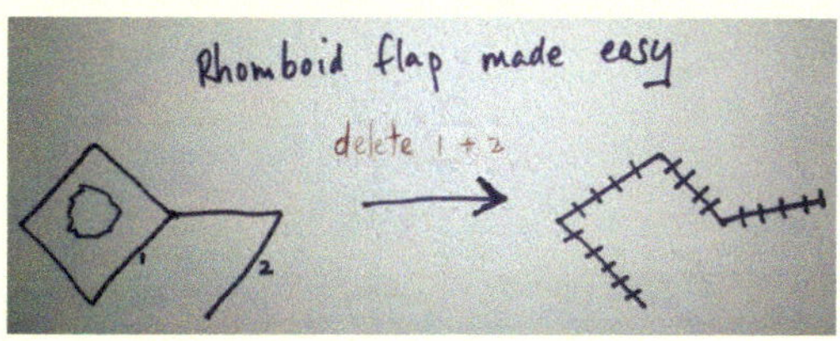

Advanced question(s)	Answer
Who first described the rhomboid flap?	• Limberg 1946

2.28 RHINOPHYMA

CLINICAL PHOTOGRAPH	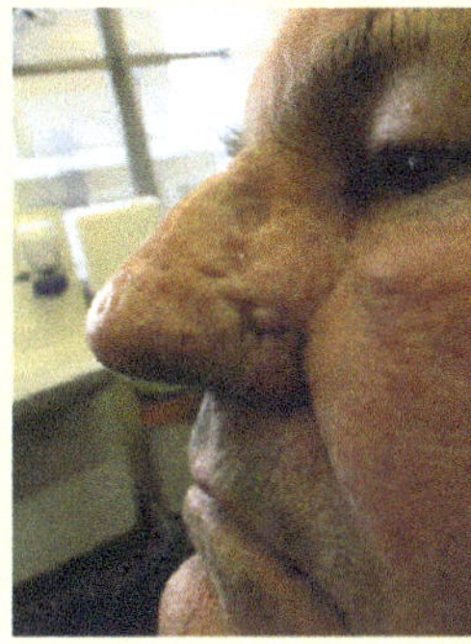

Introductory question	Answer
Describe what you see in this picture.	• This is Rhinophyma which is due to hypertrophy and hyperplasia of sebaceous glands in the skin and associated with the face mite demodex folliculorum • There is evidence of scars suggesting previous surgical intervention. • Also be aware that other cutaneous malignancies e.g. SCC/ BCC could be concealed underneath.

Competency question(s)	Answer

What causes rhinophyma?	• Unknown. • May be seen in patients with acne rosacea • Not linked with alcoholism
How would you diagnose rhinophyma?	• Clinical diagnosis • Punch biopsy (to rule out other pathologies e.g. BCC/ SCC)

Advanced question(s)	**Answer**
How would you manage a patient with rhinophyma?	• Consider referring this patient to the Dermatologist • Consider referring to a clinical psychologist for support • Varied treatment options but the principles are paring down the bulky tissue to either allow re-epithelialisation or split-skin grafting. • A variety of lasers have been used e.g. Nd:YAG, Er:YAG, Argon, carbon dioxide in a resurfacing mode (Sharplan 4 - 7 mm spot at 20 - 40W or continuous 10 - 20 W using a defocused 2 - 3mm beam). • Debulking can also be done using the microdebrider and FloSeal™ applied topically for haemostasis.

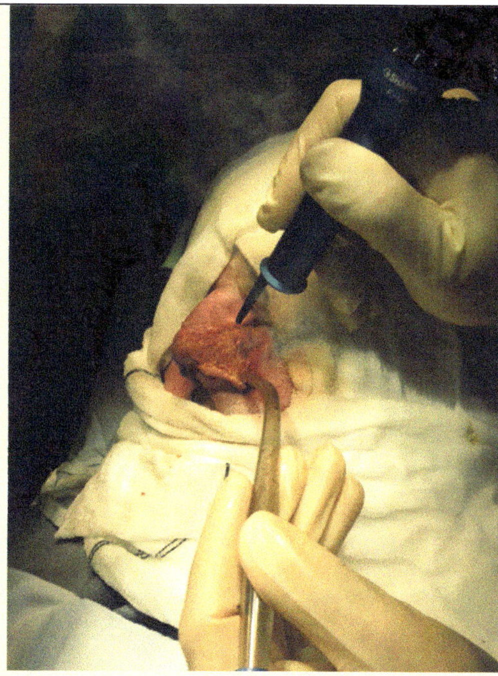

2.29 LOWER LIP SCC AND KARAPANDZIC FLAP

CLINICAL PHOTOGRAPH	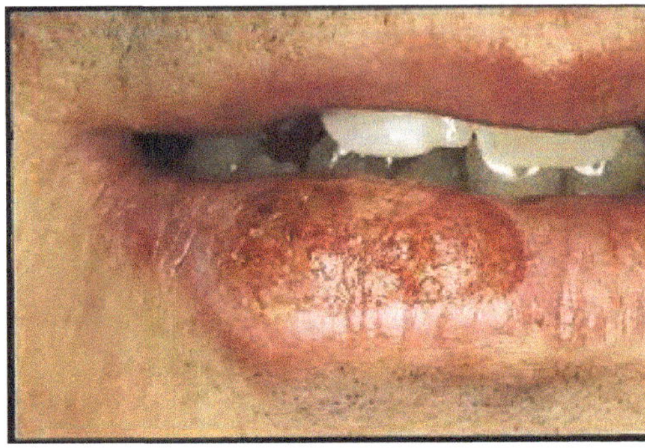

Introductory question	**Answer**
What is your differential diagnosis of the image seen above?	• BENIGN OR MALIGNANT LESION • TRAUMA, INFECTION, INFLAMATION • BCC, SCC MALIGNANT MELANOMA
Competency question(s)	**Answer**
How would you manage this patient? Biopsy comes	• History and ENT examination • If cause is not clear, I would arrange an incision or punch biopsy, which can be done under a local anaesthesia.

back as SCC. What would you do? How would you treat this lesion surgically and reconstruct the defect?	• Skin MDT • MOH surgery or excision with at least 4mm margins • Reconstruction ladder
Advanced question(s)	**Answer**
What is a Karapandzic flap?	• Karapandzic flap is rotation advancement lip flap to restore circumoral sphincter • the main disadvantage is small mouth opening

2.30 Z-PLASTY

CLINICAL PHOTOGRAPH	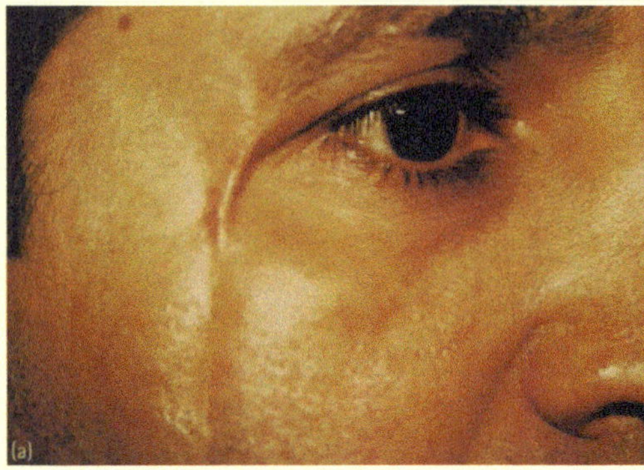

Introductory question	Answer
This 35 year old man is unhappy about the scar next to his eyes How would you deal with this problem?	• The scar needs revising; however, one should always consider if camouflaging with makeup as a option in managing scar disorder. • A Z-plasty would be the best technique to revised such as scar because lengthening is required as well as changing the direction of the scar. • A Z-plasty is an example of a transposition flap.

Competency question(s)	Answer
Show me how you would do a Z-plasty	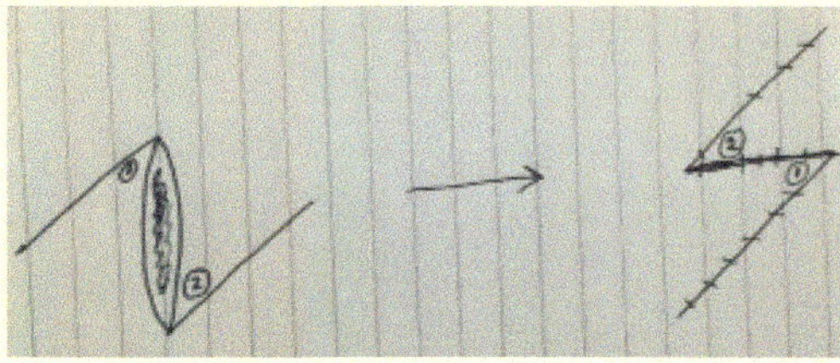 Diagram illustrating z-plasty after removal of scar tissue (*An easy way to draw before and after is to remember **Z** becomes **S**)* 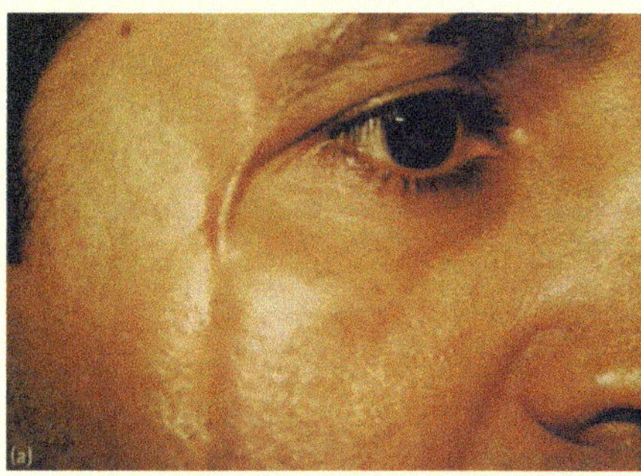 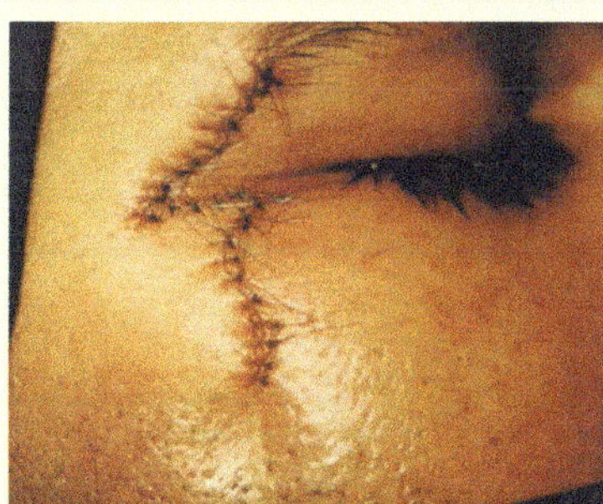
By how much is the scar lengthened?	

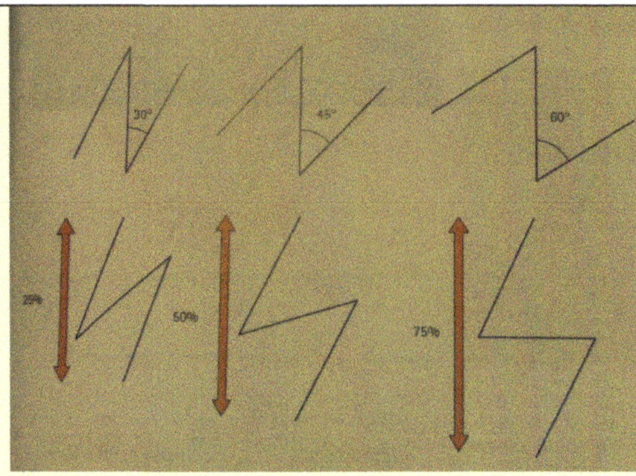

	Note that the direction of the scar and the length of the scar increase depending on the angles used; the rule is every 15 degrees there is an increase in length of 25 percent (so 30 degress/25 %; 45 degrees/50% ; 60 degrees/75% etc)
Advanced question(s)	**Answer**
What is your understanding of the reconstruction ladder?	• Level 1 – healing by 2nd intention eg concave surfaces on nose eye ears and temple (NEET vs NOCH*), primary closure, delayed primary closure • Level 2 – graft (split skin, full thickness, composite) • Level 3 – flaps (local and regional) • Level 4 - Free flaps • Level 5 – Prosthesis *Convex surfaces heal poorly by secondary intension, nose, oral, cheek helix

CHAPTER 3

Head and Neck Surgery

3.1 SALIVARY GLAND NEOPLASM

CLINICAL IMAGES	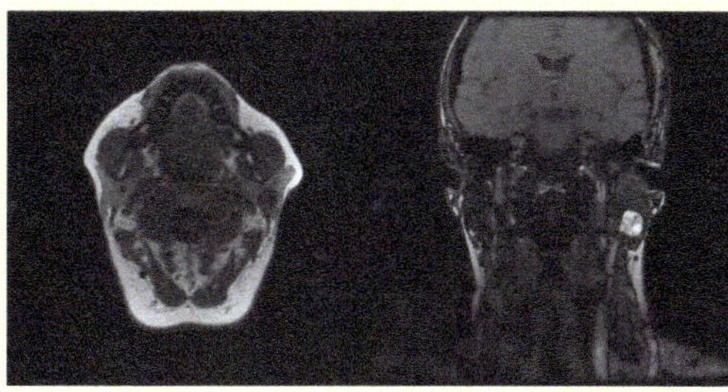

Introductory question	Answer
You have been referred a 60 year old woman with a slowly growing mass in her neck. She is otherwise completely asymptomatic. Describe what	• This is a T1-weighted MRI scan (axial and coronal). • There is around, well defined mass within the left parotid gland on axial image. This mass is bright on the coronal image post-gadolinium contrast. • There is no lymphadenopathy, erosion of the mandible or invasion of the

you see.	sternocleidomastoid muscle.
Competency question(s)	**Answer**
Based on these scans, what is your differential diagnosis?	• **Parotid neoplasm** (benign or malignant). Overall, benign parotid lesions are most common e.g. pleomorphic adenoma, Warthin's. **Intra-parotid lymph node.** This would likely be pathological and a thorough diagnostic workup is necessary, including otoscopy, and rule out any cutaneous lesions.
What clinical features are you aware of which suggests parotid gland malignancy?	• Pain, rapid growth, fixity to surrounding structures, nerve involvement or neck metastasis.
How would you manage a patient with a parotid pleomorphic adenoma?	• **Conservative.** Not unreasonable option, especially if the patient is medically unfit for surgery. Patients should be appropriately counselled on the risks of malignant change (carcinoma ex pleomorphic) and continued growth of the tumour (large tumours place the facial nerve at risk during surgery). • **Surgery**
Advanced question(s)	**Answer**
You decide to operate and during the procedure, there is tumour	• It is well documented that tumour spillage pertains to a higher rate of recurrence. Revision parotid surgery is challenging with a higher risk of trauma to the facial nerve.

spillage. Given that the pathology is benign, is this occurrence significant? What would you do in the event of tumour spillage?	• Continue with the operation. There is no evidence that any intra-operative manoeuvre decreases the risk of recurrence. Most surgeons would cover the breached tumour surface with a swab and wash the surrounding surgical site with copious amounts of saline. If the breach is small or limited to the tumour capsule, some surgeons even repair it to prevent actual spillage of neoplastic tissue into the surrounding wound. The parotid bed is again washed out at the end of the operation. • Importantly, the case should be discussed at the Head and Neck MDT to decide if post-operative radiotherapy is warranted. • These patients will require long-term follow-up.

3.2 NECK LUMP

SCENARIO **(no clinical photograph)**	A GP has referred a 30 year old man with a left neck mass, which appeared following a viral upper respiratory tract infection.

Introductory question	Answer
How would you clinically assess this patient?	• **History** • **Examination** • Think central versus lateral neck masses.
What is the likely differential diagnosis in this patient?	• **Branchial cyst** • Lymphadenopathy (reactive, infective) • Neoplastic (lymphoma, metastasis)
How would you investigate this patient?	• USS +/- FNA (first line) • CT/MRI Neck (adjuncts to diagnosis and planning of surgery)
What is the typical description given to	• Straw/ cream-colored, cloudy, low cellularity

the FNA aspirate for a brachial cyst?	
Competency question(s)	**Answer**
What is the pathogenesis of branchial cyst?	• Theories include branchial cleft remnant or trapped embryonic cells within a lymph node.
Assuming this patient has a branchial cyst, how would you manage this patient?	• **Watchful wait** – whilst it is not entirely unreasonable, the patient should be counselled that the cyst may persist or acutely enlarge following another infection causing potential airway compromise. • **Surgical excision**
Describe the images you see. CT scans in axial, coronal and saggital planes respectively. There is a low intensity mass on the left side of the neck (Level 2/3), beneath the sternocleidomastoid muscle. The mass appears to be well defined and there is no evidence of	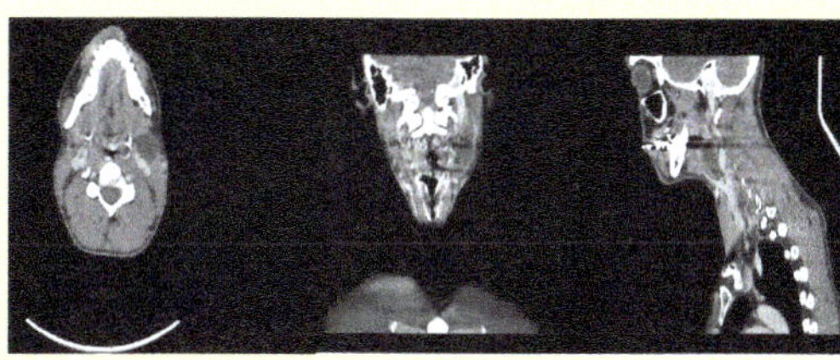

lymphadenopathy.	
Advanced question(s)	**Answer**
Would your management be any different in an older patient, say for example, aged 55 years old? How would you manage such a patient?	• Yes! An older patient presenting with a lump which appears to represent a branchial cyst on ultrasound should be regarded as having a malignancy until proven otherwise. The 'branchial cyst' could represent a cystic metastatic lymph node. • Further imaging of the neck and chest should be undertaken (if not already previously performed). Ideally the scans and FNA cytology should be discussed at a Head and Neck MDT to facilitate targeted biopsies of the upper aerodigestive tract . • If the scans remain equivocal, some units would consider a PET-CT scan which may be part of their diagnostic protocol for an unknown primary. • Otherwise, an examination under anaesthetic, multiple blind biopsies (PNS, base of tongue, pyriform fossa) and excision of the cystic mass may be reasonable. Should such an undertaking be considered, it may be worth placing the skin incision in a line for a possible neck dissection in the future.

3.3 HOARSE VOICE

SCENARIO **(followed by a clinical photograph)**	A 25 year old man presents with a hoarse voice which is getting worse. He is otherwise fit and well. However, he smokes 10 cigarettes a day and drinks socially.

Introductory question	**Answer**
What is your differential diagnosis and what procedure would you perform in clinic to make a diagnosis?	Benign or malignant cause • Benign: vocal cord nodules or cysts, nerve palsy (vagus or RLN), Papilloma. • Malignant in view of smoking and alcohol history • Fine Nasal Endoscopy examination (FNE).
Competency question(s)	**Answer**
This is what you see on FNE, how would you manage the case and what is the cause for this condition?	• This is the typical appearance of laryngeal Papilloma. • The aetiological agent is Human Papilloma Virus (HPV). • After taking a full history and examining the patient I would list the patient for

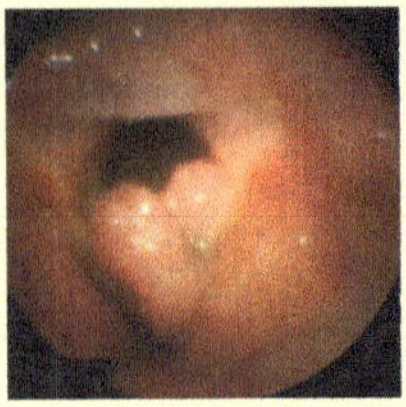	microlaryngoscopy and excision biopsy of the lesions using cold steel or a microdebrider. Care must be taken to avoid webbing in the region of the anterior commissure. • In cases of frequent reoccurrences, I would consider further surgical debridement along with adjuvant therapy such as intra-lesional cidofovir or antiviral agents eg ribavirin. • The histology is likely to show HPV subtypes HPV 6 or 11 (the latter is more aggressive).
Advanced question(s)	**Answer**
Why might the incidence of this condition decrease in the future?	• Vaccination: Gardasil offers some protection against HPV 6,11, 16 and 18 while Cervirix offers protection against subtypes 16 and 18 only.

3.4 CARCINOMA OF UNKNOWN PRIMARY (CUP)

SCENARIO (with clinical photograph)	A 56 year old male presents with a 2 month history of left neck swelling. He is otherwise fit and well. He is a smoker (15 cigarettes/day) and drinks 20 units per week. 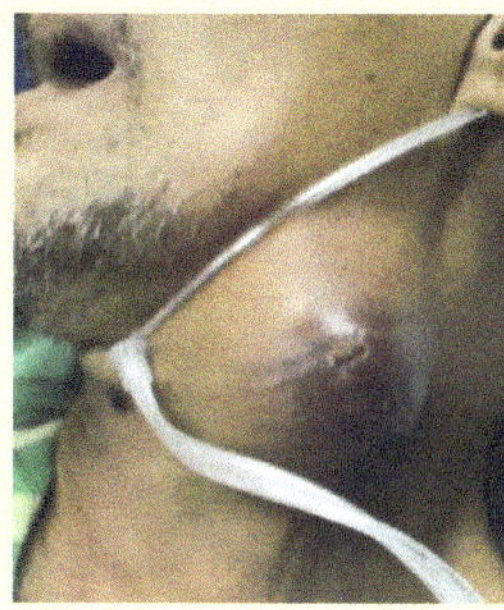

Introductory question	Answer
What is your differential diagnosis?	Malignant causes: • Secondary (metastatic neck disease) • Primary: E.g. lymphoma, submandibular/parotid gland tumour Benign causes: • Paraganglioma • Nerve sheath tumour • Laryngocele

	• Reactive/infected node i.e.TB
Competency question(s)	**Answer**
Assuming it is a metastatic node, how would you investigate the case?	• After a full history pertaining to red flag symptoms and complete otolaryngological examination including FNE, I will proceed to requesting an ultrasound-guided Fine Needle Aspiration for Cytology (FNAC). • I will also request a staging MRI scan of the head and neck as well as a CT scan of chest and upper-abdomen • If a primary is obvious on examination, I will proceed to doing a pharyngo-laryngo-oesphagoscopy with a view to obtaining a tissue diagnosis from the primary and also rule out synchronous primary disease within the upper-aerodigestive tract. • If no primary disease is detected, I will request a half-body CT-PET scan to look for a source particularly within the oropharynx and then perform panendoscopy with bilateral tonsillectomies and targeted biopsies of any site of increased activity seen on the scan.
Advanced question(s)	**Answer**
If it turns out to	• Multi-disciplinary team involvement

be an unknown primary with a single 2.5 cm level II node, how would you treat?	• This can be treated either by selective neck dissection or neck irradiation of ipsilateral levels II-IV. Since 40-55% of all metastatic neck disease arise from oropharyngeal primaries, this would provide adequate control. If extracapsular spread (ECS) is seen in the neck dissection specimen, adjuvant RT is indicated. • There is no evidence to suggest that combined modality treatment (unless evident ECS) or mucosal irradiation increases either overall survival or loco-regional control.

3.5 TONSILLAR CARCINOMA

Clinical photographs	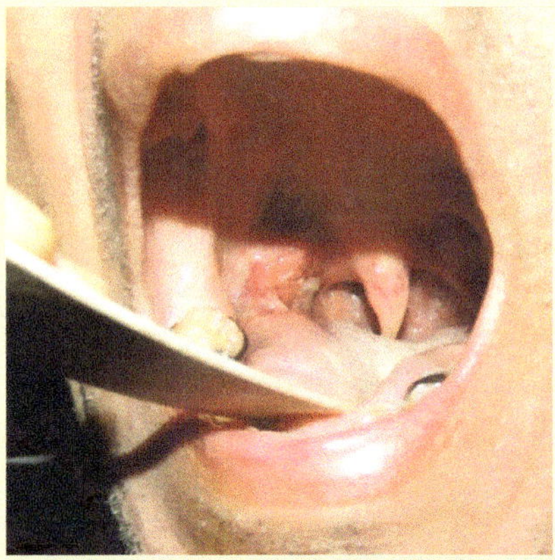 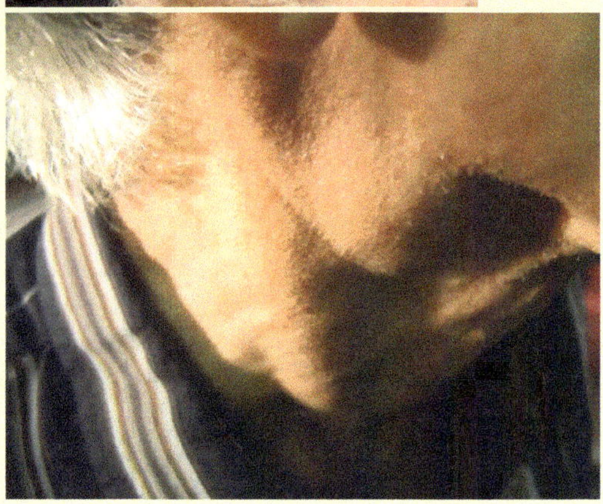

Introductory question	**Answer**
What do you see and what is your most likely diagnosis?	• Considering this is an elderly gentleman, this is most likely a right tonsillar malignancy with metastatic neck disease.
Competency question(s)	**Answer**
How would you treat it assuming it is is a T2N2bM0 SCC and patient is willing to undergo treatment?	• MDT setting • T2N2b puts this disease as a stage 3 and therefore advanced malignancy. Early malignancy (stage1-2) is treated with unimodality treatment and advanced (stage 3-4) with multimodality treatment. • Therefore, this case needs multi-modality treatment with curative intent i.e. i) Surgery followed by chemoradiotherapy (CRT) /RT alone (if chemotherapy is contra-indicated i.e age > 70 years/poor renal function) ii) CRT followed by ipsilateral neck dissection. • Surgical options include: a) ipsilateral selective neck dissection followed by chemoradiotherapy b) traditional lip split mandibulotomy with wide excision plus free flap reconstruction with bilateral selective neck dissection

	c) transoral laser/robotic-assisted resection of primary disease plus bilateral selective neck dissection.
Advanced question(s)	**Answer**
How might the HPV status affect management and outcomes?	• HPV +ve tumours have a better prognosis than if HPV-ve. • Ang *et al* NEJM 2010, demonstrated distinct stratification in prognosis based on HPV and smoking status into high risk (HPV-ve smokers), intermediate risk (HPV+ve smokers) and low-risk (HPV+ve non-smokers) tumours. • While it is not yet proven, research through De-ESCALaTE, RTOG 1016 and ECOG de-intensification studies hope to determine whether treatment for HPV +ve tumours could be de-escalated. Options could include RT in combination with Cetuximab (instead of standard CRT) or de-intensification of RT dose.

3.6 NASOPHARYNGEAL CARCINOMA

CLINICAL PHOTOGRAPH	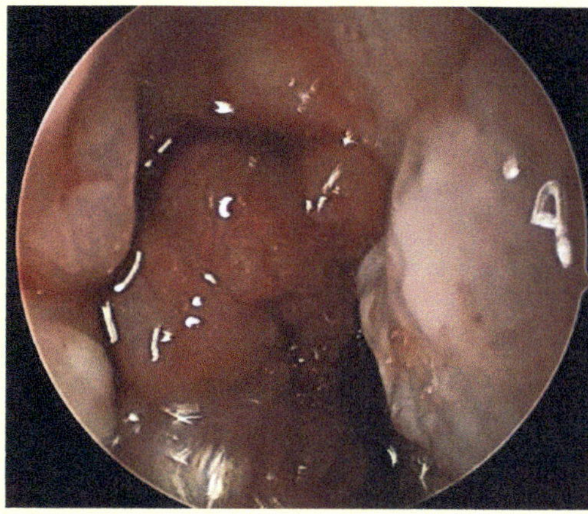

Introductory question	**Answer**
This is an endoscopic view of the nose of a 55 year old Chinese man complaining of nasal blockage, hearing loss and epistaxis. Describe what you see and tell	• There is a fleshy lesion in the posterior part of the nose consistent with either a benign process (such as adenoid hypertrophy) or a malignant lesion (such as a nasopharyngeal carcinoma) • Considering the patient is from Asia, I would be very concerned that this is a possible nasopharyngeal carcinoma.

me the most likely diagnosis.	
Competency question(s)	**Answer**
What is the incidence of NPC in Asia compared to Europe?	• 25/100,000 in SE Asia compared to 1/100,000 in Europe; Bimodal pattern (adolescent, 50-60yrs), M:F = 2:1
Why is there a higher incidence of NPC in Asia?	• Multifactorial: genetics, salted fish (nitrosamines) and EBV • EBV is particularly associated with WHO type 2 (non-keratinising SCC) and 3 (undifferentiated NPC) • WHO Type 1 NPC is keratinizing SCC
How would you investigate this patient?	• Audiogram and tympanogram • FBC, U&E, LFTs; IgA and IgG to EBV Viral capsid antigen (correlate tumour burden) • USS and FNAC neck masses • CT head neck and chest • CSF microscopy if skull base is breached • MRI if intracranial extension suspected • Consider PET

Advanced question(s)	Answer
Explain T2N2M0 classification for NPC	• T2 means that there is parapharyngeal extension of the cancer; • N2 means that there is either bilateral metastases in lymph nodes or 6cm or less in greatest dimension above the supraclavicular fossa. • M0 means there is no distant metastasis
What treatment modality would the MDT decide to use?	• In adult cases: Concurrent cisplatin or 5FU with RT • In Paediatric cases: Neoadjuvant chemo followed RT (IMRT if possible to avoid cord damage).

3.7 LARYNGEAL CARCINOMA AND NECK DISSECTION

CLINICAL PHOTOGRAPHS	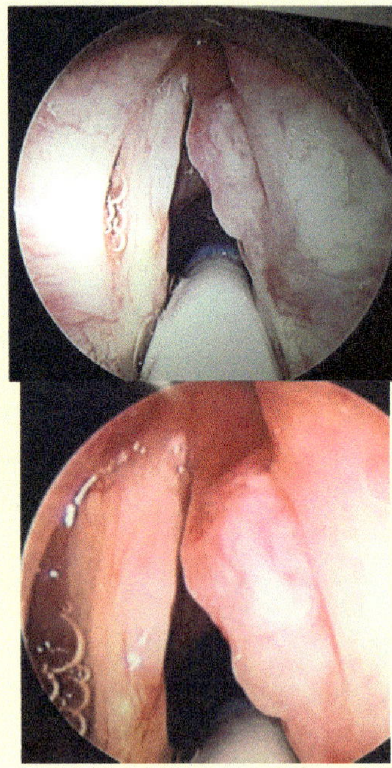

Introductory question	Answer
What is your differential diagnosis?	• Benign lesion eg granuloma, amyloid • Malignant lesion eg SCC

Competency question(s)	Answer
How would you manage this patient?	• History, examination including flexible nasendoscopy • CT neck and chest • Microlaryngoscopy and biopsy
What are the treatment options for a T1a No SCC lesion?	• Treatment options: cold steel, laser, radiotherapy
What if the CT scan shows a synchronous lesion? Which one takes priority?	• Larynx because of the greater risk of airway obstruction
What are the different types of neck dissections?	• **radical neck dissection** – removal of all cervical nodes, SMG, IJV, SCM and XI nerve • **modified radical neck dissection** – removal of levels I-V cervical nodes with preservation of one or more of 3 non-lymphatic structures (IJV, SCM and XI) • **selective neck dissection** (usually for N0 neck) 1. levels I-III for oral lesions

	2. levels II-IV for larynx and hypopharynx 3. levels II-V usually for skin tumours eg melanoma 4. level VI – for thyroid cancer • **Extended neck dissection**
Advanced question(s)	**Answer**
Why is it possible to take both IJVs during bilateral neck dissection?	• Emissary veins dilate and allow venous blood flow from the intracranial to extracranial systems.

3.8 SUPRACLAVICULAR METASTATIC SQUAMOUS CELL CARCINOMA

SCENARIO **(no clinical photograph)**	GP referral (2WW): Many thanks for urgently reviewing this 60 year old man with a 6 week history of an increasing right sided neck lump

Introductory question	Answer
What is the differential diagnosis?	• **Benign** – infective (bacterial, viral, TB), lipoma, vascular, neural • **Malignant**- primary (lymphoma), secondary (SCC from aerodigestive tract or other site eg. Chest or abdomen, bearing in mind the location of the lesion).
Competency question(s)	**Answer**
What features in the history and examination findings would help you distinguish between a benign or malignant	• **History**: Rate of growth of lump; pain; otalgia; hoarseness; dysphagia; odynophagia; weight loss; smoking; night sweats; travel abroad; haemoptysis; history of local infection of lump; history of URTI • **Examination:** neck node features – size,

cause? Assume there is a 5cm fixed lump found in the right supraclavicular fossa, with no other abnormality found on ENT examination including FNE. What investigations would you arrange? What about an incisional biopsy?	site (this can give a clue as to the possible primary site), fixity, skin involvement; neural involvement; oral cavity examination; flexible nasendoscopy of upper aerodigestive tract. • Bloods, CXR, CT scan neck and chest, USS guided FNAC. • FNAC is first choice if suspect SCC, however in younger patients with risk of lymphoma, may prefer trucut core biopsy as FNAC often not sufficient yield to make diagnosis of lymphoma. • Incisional biopsy would be a diagnostic option once SCC is excluded.
Advanced question(s)	**Answer**
FNAC confirms SCC and FNE does not demonstrate a primary lesion. What would you do?	• Aim is to find the primary site and stage the tumour. As primary site is likely to be infraclavicular, consider PET scan before panendoscopy to identify primary. If the primary is ultimately within the upper aerodigestive tract, the PET will also better direct biopsies to likely sites. Also need to undertake full staging investigations including CT scan chest/abdomen.

If the FNAC shows SCC, how would you treat the patient?	• **Treatment:** Always in conjunction with Head & Neck MDT and following full discussion with patient and relatives, taking into account patient comorbidities. - Management of the neck: Neck dissection +/- RXT depending on histological prognostic factors such as extracapsular spread, neurovascular invasion. - Management of the primary if site identified: ChemoRXT or surgery. • Management of the occult primary: Wide field RXT to likely sites or watch and wait, balancing effectiveness of treatment against morbidity from RXT.

3.9 BLACK HAIRY TONGUE

CLINICAL PHOTOGRAPH	Dorsal surface of the tongue showing taste buds 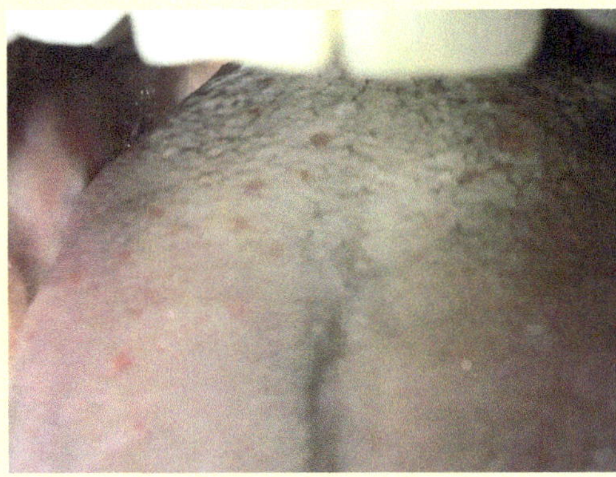

Introductory question	Answer
What are the different types of papillae found on the tongue?	• There are 4 different types of papillae present on the tongue: fungiform, filiform, foliate and circumvalate. • Generally they contain the receptors for taste (taste buds) except the filiform papillae, which are long and thin and most numerous.

<table>
<tr><th>Competency question(s)</th><th>Answer</th></tr>
<tr><td>Tell me what you know about the condition shown in this photograph?
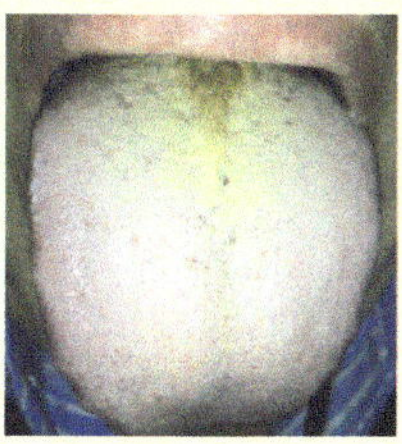</td><td><ul>
<li>Clinical photograph of the dorsal surface of the tongue consistent with the diagnosis of a black hairy tongue.</li>
<li>It is a condition of defective desquamation, hypertrophy and elongation of the filiform papillae which are present throughout the surface of the tongue.</li>
<li>It is called black hairy tongue because of keratinisation but does not have to be black in colour.</li>
<li>May be due to poor oral hygiene, low roughage diet, antibiotic usage or post-Radiotherapy.</li>
<li>It is more common in males, especially those who smoke and drink lots of tea and coffee. Also increased incidence in HIV, IV drug usage. Higher in those incarcerated.</li>
<li>The condition is mostly asymptomatic but when candidal overgrowth occurs it may lead to burning tongue syndrome (or Glossodynia).</li>
<li>The condition may be treated with brushing and or tongue scraping. Diet changes i.e. more roughage, less caffeine etc.</li>
<li>Surgery is reserved for unresponsive cases; Electrodessication, CO_2 laser,</li>
</ul></td></tr>
</table>

	scissors.
Advanced question(s)	**Answer**
How would you distinguish this condition from oral hairy leukoplakia?	• Oral hairy leukoplakia is a white patch on the side of the tongue with a hairy appearance and occurs mainly in patients who are immunocompromised (hence HIV-associated hairy leukoplakia). • It is caused by Epstein-Barr Virus (EBV) and therefore may be distintuished from black hairy tongue by punch biopsy and immunostaining for EBV.

3.10 BENIGN PAROTID LESION

SCENARIO **(clinical photograph)**	GP referral: Thank you for seeing this 67 year old man with a six month history of a swelling on the side of the face which has recently become painful. 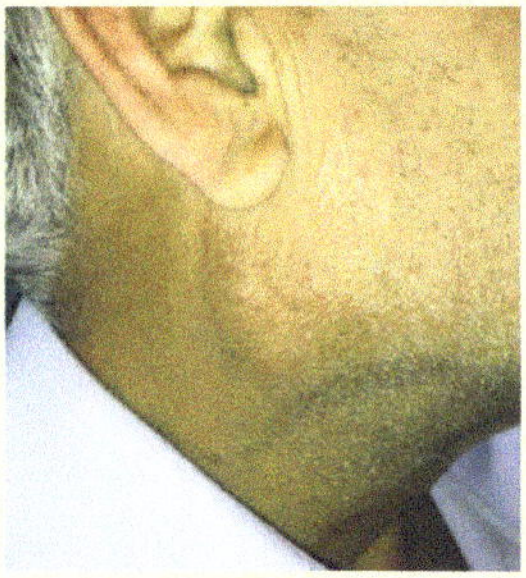

Introductory question	**Answer**
What do you see in the photograph and what is your differential diagnosis?	• This is a swelling in the upper part of the neck in the region of the parotid gland. It may represent a benign or malignant salivary or non-salivary lesion.
Competency question(s)	**Answer**
How would you manage this	• *History:* swelling constant or intermittent, relation to eating/drinking, pain, facial nerve palsy, smoking, weight

patient?	loss, medical comorbidities (dehydration, diabetes, sarcoid). • *Examination:* swelling – firm or soft; location – clench teeth (parotid or masseter); intraoral examination (Deep lobe; also Stensens and Whartons ducts, stones); neck nodes; FNE of upper aerodigestive tract (UADT). • Investigation – Ultrasound plus FNAC, MRI scan.
Assuming FNAC is suggestive of pleomorphic adenoma and you are performing a parotidectomy – describe how you would preserve the facial nerve in the surgery?	• To preserve the facial nerve (CNVII): - CNVII nerve monitor - Surgical landmarks - tympanomastoid suture, posterior belly digastric; tragal pointer - Measures to minimise bleeding: Hypotensive anaesthesia, local anaesthetic with adrenaline, head up position, gentle dissection above plane of nerve.
What would you do if the patient woke up from surgery with a VII nerve palsy?	• Postop CNVII palsy: - Wait for LA to wear off. - Is the palsy expected (i.e. if the tumour was involved with the nerve) or unexpected. If unexpected: manage any compression (eg. haematoma), consider steroids; monitor closely. - If palsy does not recover, consider nerve conduction studies for prognostic

	purposes. - May need facial reanimation techniques (CNVII grafting or repair if known to be transected, otherwise static or dynamic reanimation methods).
Advanced question(s)	**Answer**
Assume histology confirms adenoid cystic carcinoma (ACC) – explain how the cytology and histology can be so apparently incongruent?	• Pleomorphic adenoma v ACC: both are from the same cell type (from the intercalated duct) and are generally well-differentiated, hence similarities in the FNAC cytology profile.
Does this change management, compared with if histology showed a pleomorphic adenoma?	• Management – ACC needs very close and long term follow up. Due to them being slow growing and well-differentiated, distant metastases can appear years later; ensure margins clear; wider scanning including chest and brain.

3.11 MALIGNANT PAROTID LESION

CLINICAL PHOTOGRAPH	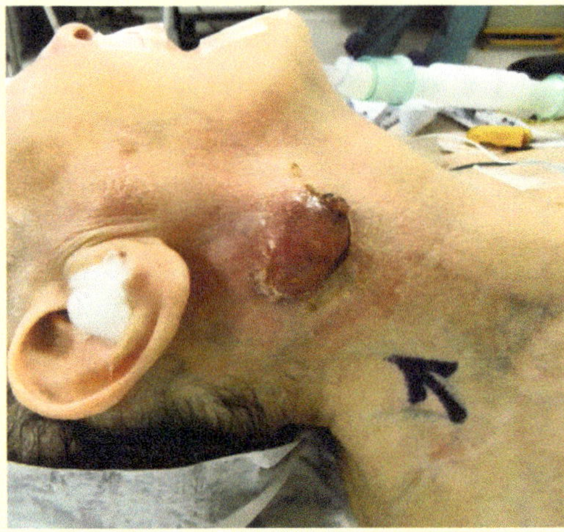

Introductory question	Answer
Describe what you see.	• Fungating lesion in the right tail of parotid region/ level 2 neck. • Further skin changes in right pre-auricular region. • Patient is under GA, on operating table site of operation marked.

Competency question(s)	Answer
What is your differential diagnosis?	• Primary cutaneous malignancy. • Fungating malignancy (lymph node, parotid).
What clinical features are you aware of which suggests parotid gland malignancy?	• Pain, rapid growth, fixed to surrounding structures, nerve involvement or neck metastasis.
How would you assess this patient in clinic and what investigations would you have requested for?	• Ultrasound guided FNAC is recommended for all salivary tumours and cytology should be reported by an experienced expert histopathologist. • Some units undertake MRI neck and CT chest to stage the disease. • It is imperative to discuss the patient at a head and neck MDT.
What is the role of frozen section in diagnosing parotid neoplasms?	• Accurate diagnosis is often difficult and false negative rates are significant; hence frozen section should not be relied on except for establishing excision margins.
Apart from parotidectomy, how will you manage a patient as seen in the	• Neck dissection is recommended in all cases of malignant parotid tumours except for low grade small tumours. Therapeutic neck dissection is indicated for lymph node involvement. Elective

picture?	neck dissection is indicated for high-stage and clinically high-grade disease such as high-grade adenocarcinoma, carcinoma ex-pleomorphic adenoma, squamous cell carcinoma, high-grade mucoepidermoid and undifferentiated carcinoma. The following factors are indications for post operative radiotherapy: • microscopic residual disease. • adenoid cystic tumours. • aggressive undifferentiated tumours. • large tumours "4cm rule".
Advanced question(s)	**Answer**
How would you manage the facial nerve in this patient?	• As a general principle, if the facial nerve function is normal pre-operatively then every attempt to preserve facial nerve function should be made during Parotidectomy. If the facial nerve is divided intra-operatively, then immediate microsurgical repair (with an interposition graft if required) should be considered. • See ENTUK Head and Neck Cancer: Multidisciplinary Management Guidelines, 2011.

3.12 VOCAL CORD DYSPLASIA/EARLY GLOTTIC SCC

SCENARIO **(no clinical photograph)**	GP referral (2 week wait): Thank you for seeing this 50 year old patient with a two month history of hoarseness.

Introductory question	Answer
How would you manage this patient?	• **History**: hoarseness – questions primarily focussed at assessing risk factors (smoking & alcohol, weight loss, occupation, history of thyroid problems, acid reflux); also is hoarseness persistent or intermittent; referred otalgia; haemoptysis; aspiration; associated dysphagia; odynophagia. • **Examination:** full neck examination for cervical lymphadenopathy; examination of oral cavity; FNE of larynx and pharynx. • **Investigations:** baseline blood tests including FBC; TFTs; CXR; further investigations to be guided following clinical assessment.
Competency question(s)	**Answer**
What is your	• **Benign**: chronic laryngitis,

differential diagnosis?	laryngopharyngeal reflux, benign growths (nodule, polyp, cyst, sulcus, papillomata). • **malignant**: dysplasia; malignant lesion (SCC).
How would you make a diagnosis?	• Microlaryngoscopy + Biopsy
Biopsy shows dysplasia – what do you do?	• Re-biopsy if biopsy and clinical suspicion do not correlate well (i.e. do not trust a negative histology). If representative – lifestyle advice (stopping smoking, reduce alcohol), regular follow up to ensure no progression.
If SCC is confirmed, what are the relative merits of Transoral Laryngeal Surgery (TOLS) versus radiotherapy (RXT)?	• **TOLS v Radiotherapy**: Local control: similar survival rates for T1, evidence suggests TOLS associated with worse results in T1b rather than T1a lesions but rates similar for radiotherapy. For T2 – poor data available for TOLS so far, RXT 70-75% 5 year survival. Overall impression: probably finely balanced decision. Surgery one off and more convenient, however consider perioperative risks in patients with comorbidities. Voice: radiotherapy affects whole larynx regardless of tumour size, whereas effects on voice with surgery are dependent on size and depth of lesion. Consensus is that surgery is worse especially if anterior commissure involved and with larger tumours. Results on

	voice are equal for small T1a lesions. Chance of requiring eventual total laryngectomy (TL): Similar for T1a lesions however treated; for T1b marginal increased chance of eventual TL if radiotherapy was the primary modality of treatment rather than TOLS; for T2 eventual TL rates lower with TOLS due to possibility for multiple TOLS salvage.
Advanced question(s)	**Answer**
If radiotherapy is given and there is a biopsy-proven recurrence after 2 years, what would your management be?	• Initial assessment as above with particular attention paid to excluding a synchronous second (usually lung) primary. • ***Treatment:*** TOLS if lesion amenable depending on staging; RXT if TOLS performed first; consider TL if fixed cords or if lesion not suitable for TOLS.

3.13 HPV AND OROPHARYNGEAL LESION

CLINICAL PHOTOGRAPHS	
	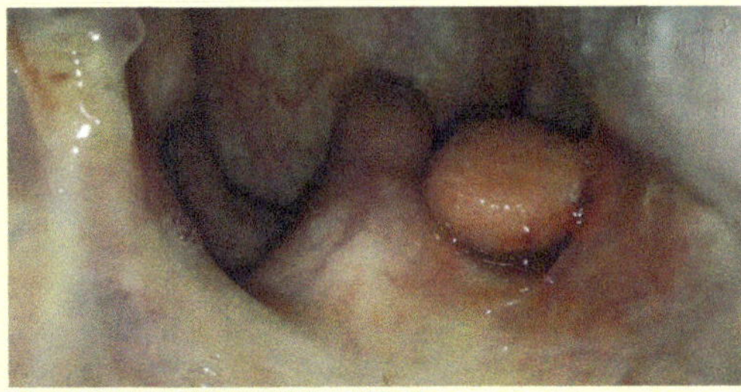 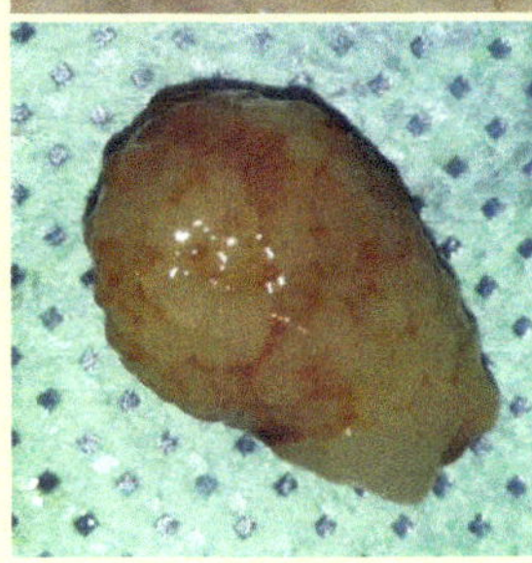

Introductory question	Answer
Describe the clinical photographs.	On the left is a clinical photograph showing a unilateral lesion in the right upper pole of the tonsillar fossa. The lesion is approximately twice the size of the uvula and has a mulberry-like appearance. The specimen is shown in the right photograph. Part of the left tonsil is visible and appears to be normal.

Competency question(s)	Answer
What is the most likely diagnosis of the lesion and tell me about the possible aetiology?	• Oral papilloma caused by HPV. • HPV 16 and 18 as associated with oropharyngeal carcinoma (tonsil and tongue base)
Tell me about HPV virus	• Small double stranded DNA virus • Most common sexually transmitted virus • Wide range of sequelae (mild disease to high-grade squamous lesions) • Mild Disease • Genital warts • Anal warts • Cervical dysplasia • Severe Disease: • Carcinomas of the cervix, vagina, vulva, anus and penis. • Non-genital types associated with warts on hands, feet etc • Over 120 subtypes
How is the virus detected?	• Method not Standardised • Direct Detection of HPV Subtype DNA is possible with PCR or in-situ hybridisation but this is very expensive

	• Immunohistochemistry for P16, a surrogate marker,, is cheaper 100% Sensitive, 79% specific. • 7% discordant rate between PCR and P16
Advanced question(s)	**Answer**
Do you think boys should also be vaccinated with HPV VACCINE?	In view of the apparent increase in incidence of HPV related oropharyngeal carcinoma in young adults, the answer is probably, Yes. Gardasil offers some protection against HPV 6,11, 16 and 18 while Cervirix offers protection against subtypes 16 and 18 only.

3.14 FACIAL PAIN

SCENARIO (no clinical photograph)	A 45 year old business woman attends your clinic complaining of facial pain.

Introductory question	Answer
What is your differential diagnosis?	• Pain may be arising from any of the multiple systems in the head and neck region such as the nervous system, rhinological system, otological system, dentition and TMJ, vascular system or ophthamological system.
Competency question(s)	**Answer**
Tell me about neurological pain?	• The four main types of neurological head pain are migraine, cluster headache, tension headache and trigeminal neuralgia. • ***Migraine*** affects about 10-15% of population and is thought to involve a trigeminovascular mechanism. It may be triggered by stress, menstruation, dietary intake (tyramine). 10% display aura

	(visual, limb or face dysaesthesia, mood change). Aura precedes pain by 10-60 mins. Throbbing unilateral pain that spreads. Photophobia, phonophobia and nausea may last 4-72 hours. Patients are often pain free between attacks. Treatment: Antiemetics, Analgesics, Ergotamine – can abort impending attack, Sumatriptan (5-HT1 agonist) given subcutaneously can abort attack, Prevention by avoiding precipitants, or trial use of beta blocker, pizotifen or methysergide. • ***Cluster headaches*** occur 1-8 times/day, each attack lasts 15 mins – 3 hours and may go on for 3-12 weeks. Patients can be symptom-free for up to 1.5 years. The deep throbbing severe headache often wakes the patient up. The headache is associated with parasympathetic overdrive such as nasal congestion, injected conjunctiva and ptosis and may be confused with allergic rhinitis. Exercise with increased sympathetic activity (eg pacing up and down) is helpful in relieving symptoms, other forms of treatment includes oxygen therapy (cerebral vasoconstriction), ergotamine, sphenopalatine ganglion LA block. • ***Tension headache*** is usually a dull aching pain which may be unilateral or bilateral. There are associated with specific trigger points in muscles such as sternocleidomastoid, trapezius, temporalis and pterygoids. Tension

	headache is linked to stress and therefore relaxation is therapeutic. • ***Trigeminal neuralgia*** is a sharp short stabbing pain in the distribution of one or more of the three branches of the trigeminal nerve. The pain occurs in response to innocuous stimuli. It is due to local demyelination of trigeminal root entry zone. This may be caused by compression by a small vein or artery in posterior cranial fossa. Treatment includes carbamazepine, gabapentin alcohol/Glycerin/Radiofrequency ablation to the trigeminal ganglion. Surgical decompression of vascular loop via a posterior fossa craniotomy is rarely required.
Advanced question(s)	**Answer**
Have you heard about post-herpetic neuralgia?	• This refers to neuropathic pain following acute herpes virus infection. • It is usually a burning pain, occasionally throbbing • The mechanism involves a modulating effect of large calibre nerve fibres (proprioceptive) at the dorsal root entry zone. • It can be treated with neuropathic agents Amitriptylline, Carbamazepine or Gabapentin. TENS, Acupuncture and Capsaicin ointment have been used.

3.15 PHARYNGEAL POUCH

SCENARIO **(followed by clinical images)**	A 74 year old man has been referred to you by his GP with a 6 month history of progressive dysphagia.

Introductory question	**Answer**
How would you assess him?	• History focusing on the onset of dysphagia, type (solids, fluids), weight loss, associated symptoms (pain, hoarseness, neck lumps, odynophagia). • Clinical examination, including fiberoptic endoscopy to rule out neoplasm.
Competency question(s)	**Answer**
On further questioning, the patient also describes post-prandial regurgitation of food and weight loss. Apart from endoscopic	• Zenker's diverticulum or pharyngeal pouch. • Differential: Oesophageal stricture, severe reflux disease/ hiatus hernia.

evidence of reflux, clinical examination was unremarkable. What is your differential diagnosis?	
How would you investigate this patient?	• Water soluble contrast, or Barium swallow.
Describe what you see. 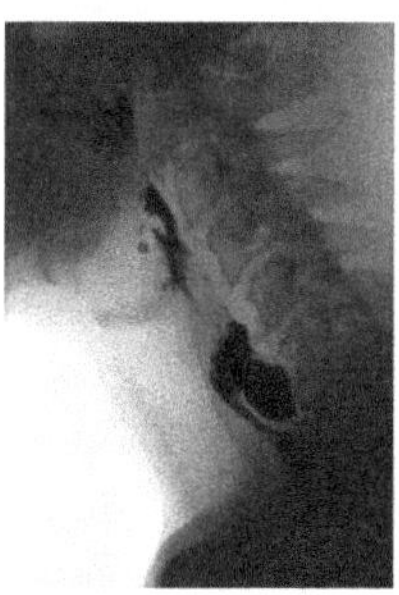	• Barium swallow image demonstrating a pharyngeal pouch. There is no evidence of a filling defect within the pouch or aspiration on this image. A full series of images would be required for confirmation.
What is a pharyngeal pouch?	• Also known as Zenker's diverticulum, it is a pulsion diverticula herniation through Killian's dehiscence (or Killian's triangle) above the cricopharyngeus muscle, between the oblique and transverse constrictor muscles of the pharynx.
How would you manage this	• Appreciating that many patients with pharyngeal pouch are elderly, an

patient?	anaesthetic opinion is needed to ensure that they are medically fit for a general anaesthetic. Endoscopic stapling is now an established technique in the UK. NICE guidance (2003) also recommend that sub-specialisation within ENT departments should occur for this procedure. • A recent literature review (Leong et al., 2012) of outcomes from UK departments reported that 92.3% (540 out of 585) were successfully stapled. Forty-five (7.7%) procedures were abandoned intra-operatively. The most common reason was difficulty assessing a small pouch. The majority of patients (92%) had resumed oral intake by the second post-operative day. Most patients (87%) were discharged by the second post-operative day. Outcomes were good with over 90% reporting resolved or significantly improved symptoms.
Advanced question(s)	**Answer**
Assuming you have successfully stapled the pouch, what are your post-operative instructions?	• Day case pharyngeal pouch stapling is not currently routine UK practice. Minor complications included dental trauma, transient hoarseness and sore throat may cause delayed resumption of oral intake. Given that many of these patients are elderly, they will require in-patient care and close observation in the immediate post-operative period.

	• The most feared complication following this procedure is perforation. The UK review (Leong et al., 2012) reported an overall perforation rate of 4.8%. The patient needs to be regularly monitored for retrosternal pain, tachypnoea, tachycardia, pyrexia and odynophagia.
What do you see on this lateral neck x-ray? 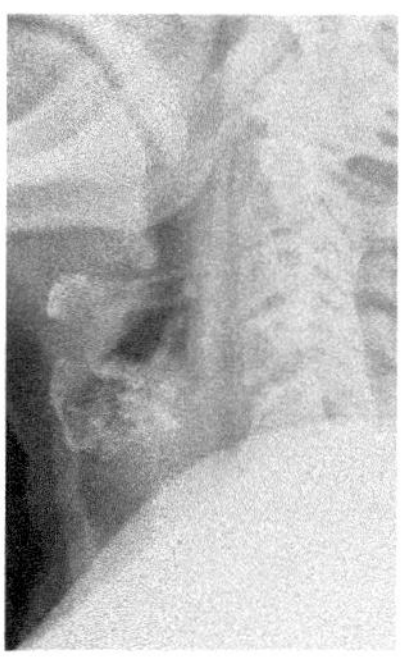	• A linear gas shadow with pre-vertebral swelling (normally C2-4 soft tissue thickness 7mm max) and straightening of the normal lordosis is typical of a perforation of the oesophagus.
How would you manage a perforated pharyngngeal pouch?	• This is an ENT emergency as delayed management may lead to serious sequelae such as mediastinitis. The patient needs to be kept nil by mouth and resuscitated as necessary. Expedient return to theatre should be planned and involvement of another senior head and neck surgeon should also be considered. • Repair of the perforation is undertaken as an external approach (left side of neck). The patient will require intravenous antibiotics, a nasogastric feeding tube and prophylactic reflux treatment.

3.16 PARAPHARYNGEAL MASS

SCENARIO **(with a clinical photograph)**	This 21-year old girl presents with a history of right neck swelling of 2 years, progressively increasing in size. Otherwise fit and well. 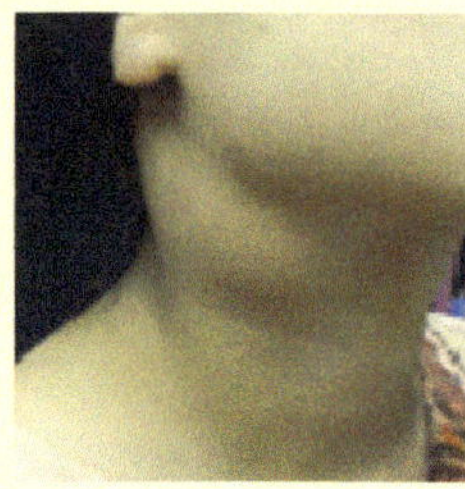

Introductory question	Answer
What are your differentials?	• Branchial cyst • Lymphadenopathy • Parapharyngeal mass
How is the parapharyngeal space divided?	• The parapharyngeal space is divided into 2 parts by the fascial condensation called aponeurosis of Zuckerkandl and Testut, joining the styloid process and tensor veli palatine muscle which arises by a flat lamella from the scaphoid fossa (of the medial pterygoid plate) from the sphenoid spine and from the lateral wall

Assuming that this is a parapharyngeal space tumour arising from the post-styloid compartment, what would be your differentials?	of the cartilage of the Eustachian tube. • Schwannoma • Paraganglioma • Neurofibroma
Competency question(s)	**Answer**
How would you manage this patient?	**History** – duration, mass effect, local neurology, FH, symptoms of excess catecholamines **Examination** - inspect mass, palpation, pulsation, bruit, inspect oral cavity for medialization **Investigation** CT scan of neck to assess mass, then proceed for FNAC if it is not vascular in origin MRI may be able to give a radiological diagnosis but may not be able to show skull-base erosion. Proceed to surgical excision if required following discussion at appropriate MDT. If paraganglioma suspected will need endocrine review +/- genetics referral.

Advanced question(s)	Answer
What are the suprahyoid spaces marked out on the MR images?	
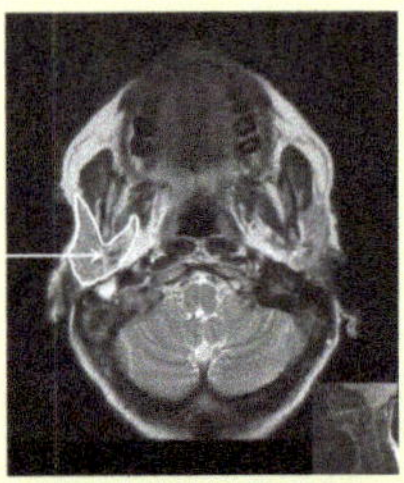	• Parotid space
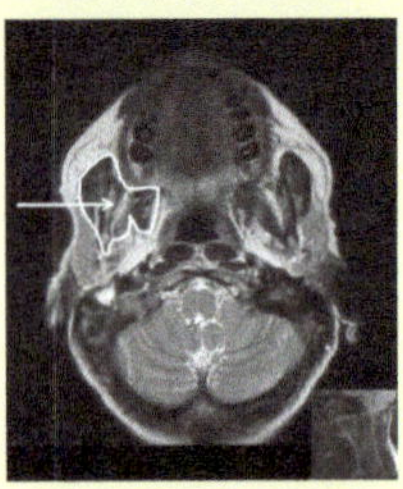	• Masticater space
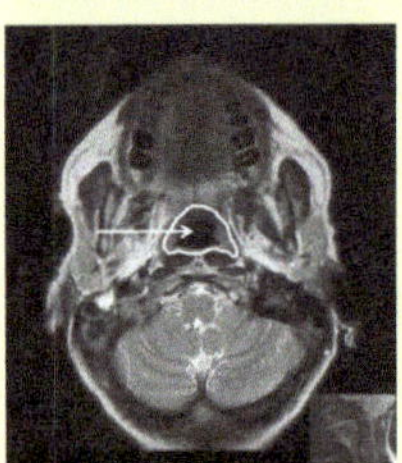	• Pharyngeal mucosal space

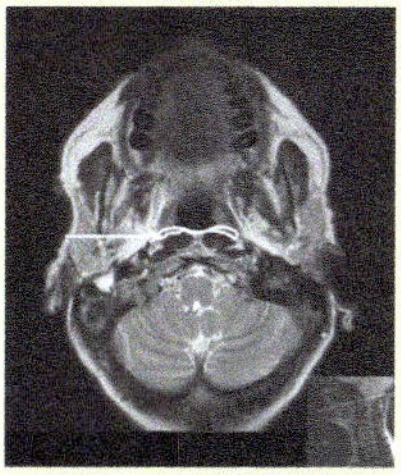	• retropharyngeal space
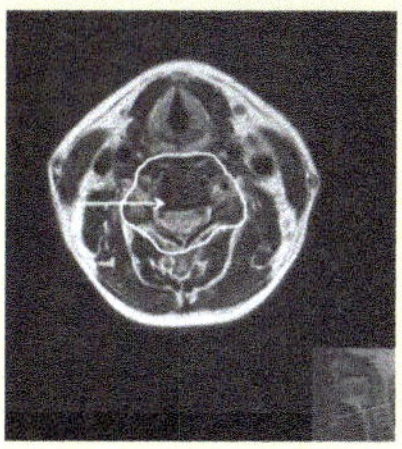	• peri-vertebral space

3.17 HEMI-TONGUE ATROPHY

CLINICAL PHOTOGRAPH	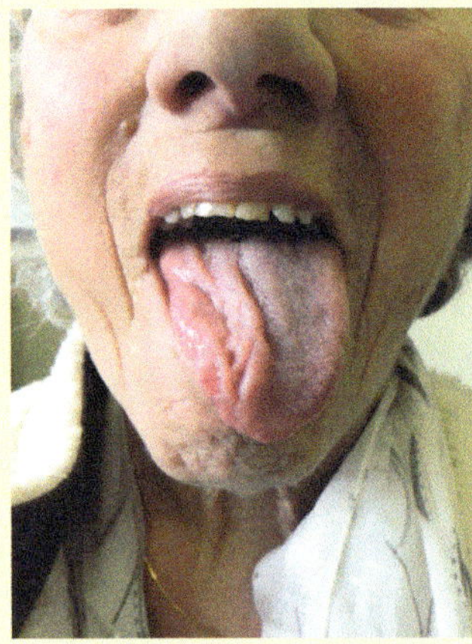
Introductory question	**Answer**
This 65-year old lady appears at the head and neck clinic for routine follow-up. Describe what you see.	• **Obvious:** Hemitongue (right) atrophy with loss of bulk and natural contours, smooth appearance (loss of papillae). • **Less obvious**: tongue fasciculation, deviation towards the side affected. Patient's own teeth! • **Not obvious**: visible scars, facial palsy, lesions on the face
What other clinical signs might you expect	• Dysarthria • Oral/ tongue ulcers due to poor deglutition

in this patient?	• Evidence of worn dentition (contralateral molars) • Neck scar, free flap etc. • Palpable neck lump
Competency question(s)	**Answer**
What is the pathophysiology of this condition?	• Hypoglossal nerve palsy (cranial nerve XII)
What may have caused the hemitongue atrophy in this patient?	• Excision of CN XII was part of a wider oncologic resection e.g. adenoid cystic carcinoma of the submandibular gland • Iatrogenic e.g. submandibular gland excision for sialolithiasis • Hypoglossal canal: schwannoma, meningioma, metastasis, spread of nasopharyngeal carcinoma, large glomus jugulare (grown into the hypoglossal canal) • Central causes: vascular e.g. thrombosis of the vertebral artery, motor neurone disease, syringobulbia

Advanced question(s)	Answer
How would you locate the hypoglossal nerve intra-operatively?	• Medial to the posterior belly of the digastric muscle. The nerve becomes exposed when the digastric is retracted superiorly. • Superiorly, the nerve emerges from the hypoglossal canal at the skull base, between the internal jugular vein and internal carotid artery. • The nerve turns anteriorly over the carotid and as it does, gives off the ansa cervicalis.
If this patient was being seen at the skull base clinic following excision of an acoustic neuroma, how would you account for the hemitongue atrophy seen here?	• The patient may have suffered facial nerve palsy as a consequence of acoustic neuroma excision. • A hypoglossal - facial nerve anastamosis is a recognised method of reanimating facial paralysis. A House-Brackman grade IV can be expected as best outcome.

3.18 CERVICAL MYCOBACTERIAL LYMPHADENITIS (SCROFULA)

SCENARIO (and Clinical photograph)	This 27 year old HIV positive patient presents with a **painless** neck lump that has be getting bigger over the last 6 months. It does not move with swallowing or tongue protrusion. 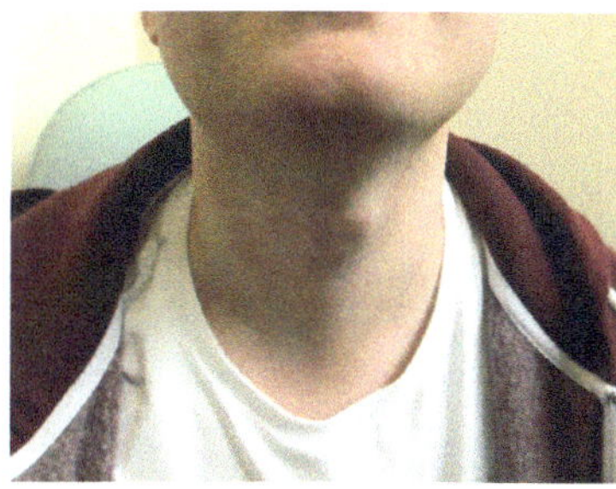 **Figure 3.18** Clinical photo showing a painless neck lump

Introductory question	Answer
What is your differential diagnosis?	• This patient may be immunocompromised and therefore at an increased risk of infectious, so an infection would be high on my list of differential diagnosis. I would also consider a neoplastic lesion.

	• So my differential diagnosis would be: 1. infections, including Tuberculous mycobacteria 2. Non-tuberculous (atypical) mycobacteria (NTM) 3. Metastatic SCC or NPC 4. Papillary thyroid carcinoma 5. Lymphoma
Competency question(s)	**Answer**
How would you attempt to make a definitive diagnosis?	• Ultrasound scan and FNAC • FNAC including Ziehl Neelsen stain for acid fast bacteria in tuberculous mycobacteria • Culture of NTM using specific growth and staining techniques
Advanced question(s)	**Answer**
Where is the commonest site for TB other than the lungs?	• The neck is the commonest site of extrapulmonary manifestation of tuberculosis. • Furthermore cervical mycobacterial lymphadenitis tends to be unilateral, with a predilection for nodes in the posterior triangle (51percent) and deep upper cervical (48 percent). • In the case of *mycobacteria tuberculosis*:

Tell How would you treat this patient?	**Multi-drug therapy** for mycobacteria tuberculosis infection (this may include pyrazinamide, isoniazid, ethambutol, rifampicin and streptomycin ('PIERS'). Note that during therapy new or existing cervical nodes may enlarge but this is not indicative of failure as it is only transient. • In the case of *non-tuberculous mycobacteria*: **Surgical excision**.

3.19 PSEUDOMEMBRANOUS COLITIS (*C.Diff* infection)

SCENARIO **(no clinical photograph)**	A 66 year old patient underwent an uneventful neck dissection. He was discharged 3 days later with 7 day course of oral Co-amoxiclav because of aspiration at the time of induction of anaesthesia. Four days later, he developed non-bloody foul smelling diarrhoea, fever, fatigue, loss of appetite and severe abdominal pain.

Introductory question	Answer
What do you think is the cause of his symptoms?	• A infective process affecting the gastro-intestinal system • In view of the antibiotic, I would consider Pseudomembranous Colitis. • MRSA is also a possibility
Competency question(s)	**Answer**
How would you manage this patient?	• Full history and examination • Admit the patient under joint care with Infectious Disease team • Send bloods for blood culture, haematological and biochemical profiles

	and resusitate patient as required • Stool sample for *C. Difficile* toxin • Stop co-amoxiclav • Rx Metronidazole +/- oral vancomycin (risk of vancomycin resistant *Enterococcus*) • Faecal transplant for refractory cases
Advanced question(s)	**Answer**
Tell me about infection control in your hospital with regards to *C.Difficile* infection.	• Isolation eg side room with own toilet • Barrier nursing • Hand washing • Own toilet in room

3.20 REINKE's OEDEMA

SCENARIO	A 45 year old woman smoker complains that her voice is becoming masculine and her friends can't recognised her on the phone anymore.

Introductory question	**Answer**
What is going through your mind?	• The history suggests Reinke's oedema of the vocal folds. • I would also be thinking of a neoplastic process since she is a smoker.
Competency question(s)	**Answer**
Which other conditions are associated with Reinke's oedema?	• Voice Abuse • Reflux • Hypothyroidism
What would you do next?	• After a taking a full history, I would proceed to examine the larynx with a flexible nasendoscope.

Draw a cross section of the vocal fold showing the various layers and Reinke's space	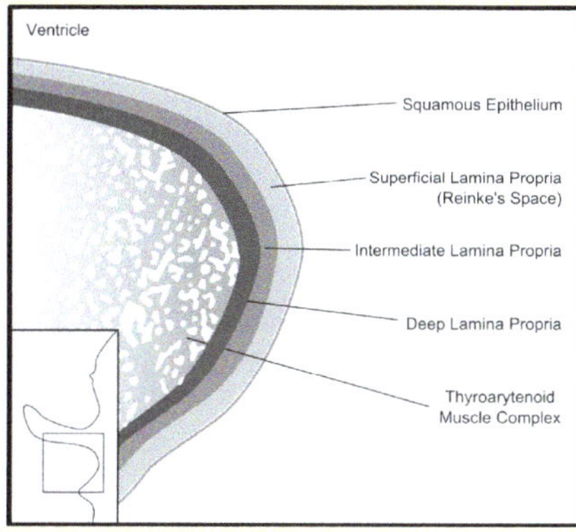
What treatment would you offer?	• Surgery only if suspicion of CANCER or AIRWAY compromise • Lateral cordotomy and suction or laser vaporization • Stop smoking • SALT
Advanced question(s)	**Answer**
Is the surgery easy or difficult?	• Difficult (arm chair surgery)
Have you ever seen Reinke's oedema in a man?	• No

3.21 RADIOTHERAPY AND SIDE EFFECTS

CLINICAL PHOTOGRAPH	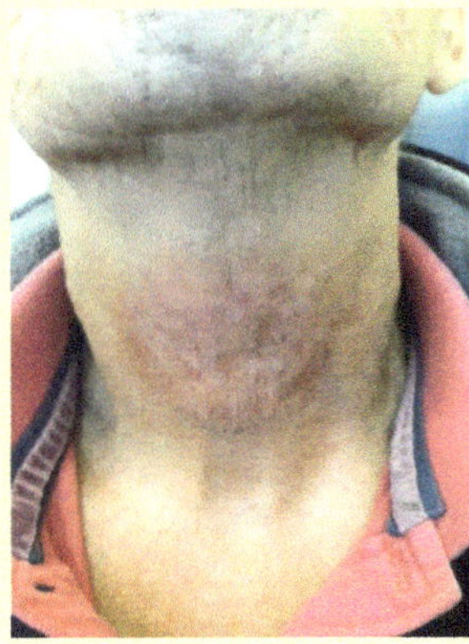

Introductory question	**Answer**
Describe the clinical photo.	• Clinical photograph of the neck showing erythema anteriorly in the region of the larynx. • The may represent radiotherapy changes or thyroiditis
Competency question(s)	**Answer**
What are the other side effects	**Acute:**

of radiotherapy	• Skin: erythema; desquamation; tanning; loss of hair follicles; sweat/sebaceous gland dysfuntion • GI: Loss of taste; salivary dysfunction; mucositis; N+D+V • Bone marrow suppression • Lung pneumonitis **Long term:** • Neck: fibrosis • Jaw: fibrosis, reduced mouth opening • Lymphatic: Lymphoedema • Wounds: delayed healing • Skin: telangectasias, ulceration leading to ORN • Salivary: xerostomia (amifostine through treatment, pilocarpine after); dental disease • CNS: transient radiation myelopathy; transverse myelitis (Lhermittes) • Endocrine: hypothyroisim, GH deficiency • Eye: cataracts, retinitis, keratitis(dry eye) • Ears: OME; SNHL • **2nd malignancy**

Advanced question(s)	Answer
How does radiotherapy works?	• Ionizing radiation interacts with water/oxygen to form free radicals which breaks dsDNA with the loss of cells reproductive capacity • Cancer cells have reduced ability to repair damage – thus selective • Normal cells produce p53 prolong 'S' stage and allow more time for DNA repair).

3.22 SCC TONGUE

SCENARIO (followed by a clinical photograph)	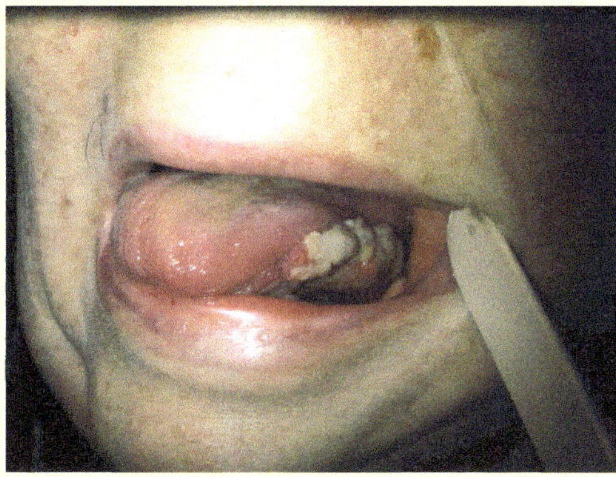

Introductory question	Answer
Tell me about this clinical photo?	• Clinical photograph showing an exophytic lesion of the left lateral surface of the tongue. • The appearance is most consistent with a malignant lesion such as squamous cell carcinoma (the 2nd commonest oral cancer); histological confirmation would be required after full history and examination.
Competency	**Answer**

question(s)	
What are the risk factors associated with SCC tongue?	• Alcohol, smoking, Human Papilloma Virus (HPV) infection (for tonsil and tongue base mainly), previous radiotherapy, betel nut chewing, sharp teeth and spicy food.
What are the treatment options?	• Conservative (if patient terminally ill with other co-morbidity) • Surgical excision with neck dissection if indicated • Chemoradiotherapy • Palliative treatment • Oral cancer is mainly treated with surgery, occasionally radiotherapy may be used. Defect may be reconstructed with a free flap such as radial forearm, anterior thigh or rectus abdominis if bulk is needed. Work up usually involves OPG, MRI oral cavity and neck, CT chest as well as EUA and biopsy.
Which staging system is used for tongue cancer?	• Panendoscopy and CT chest are important for possible synchronous lesions. • The tumour is staged by the TNM classification: T1: tumour ≤ 2cm

	T2: 2cm < tumour ≤ 4cm T3: tumour > 4cm T4: tumour invading into adjacent structures
Advanced question(s)	**Answer**
How would you deal with a N0 neck?	• Basic rule is to treat any patient whose risk of occult mets is greater than 20 percent: Metastatic risk for floor of mouth (25%), Tongue (60%), Base of tongue (55%), Buccal mucosa / Retromolar region (20%), Tonsil (36%), Aryepiglottic Fold (30%); Piriform sinus (65%). • In general cavity tumours with depth >3mm have higher risk of occult mets (>20%) • If surgery is proceeding for the primary lesion then a neck dissection should be done as it allows for histopathological staging. • Otherwise RT to primary lesion and neck • Regional recurrence of pathological N0 neck is 1.9 percent.

3.23 VOCAL PROCESS GRANULOMA

CLINICAL PHOTOGRAPH	This is an endoscopic view of the larynx in an intubated patient. 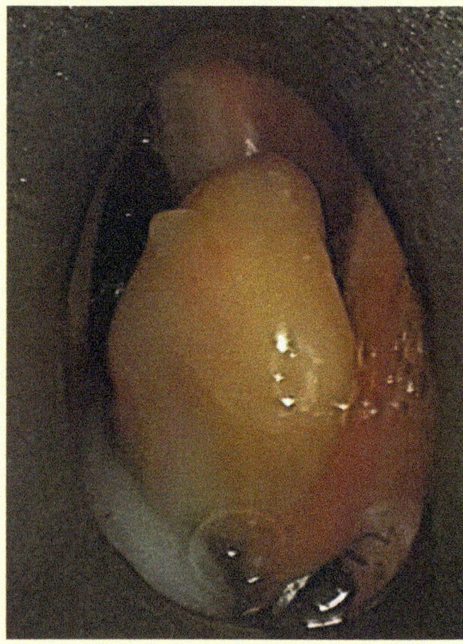

Introductory question	Answer
Describe what you see and tell me your differientials.	• A fleshy polypoidal lesion of the right hemilarynx. It is difficult to see where it is attached. • This may represent a polyp or vocal process granuloma. Other less likely

	differientials includes SCC, TB, hsitoplasmosis, coccidiomycos, blastomycosis, Wegeners, syphilis, leprosy, Crohns
Competency question(s)	**Answer**
Tell me more about vocal process granuloma.	• Uncommon benign lesions commonly centered on the vocal process of the arytenoid • Evolve from repeated insults to mucosa overlying fragile thin perichondrium (can be mehanical, inflammatory or both). • Initial ulceration leads to necrosis. • Granulomatous reaction to repaeted trauma or acid reflux • Tends to occur in male professional voice users or in females post intubation • Patients may present with chronic cough, throat clearing, hoarseness, Globus, sore throat, dyspnoea, haemoptysis

Advanced question(s)	Answer
How is the condition treated?	• Surgery: laser or cold steel – no randomised control trials regarding removal or leaving associated cartilageleave cartilage • Voice therapy – target breath control, elevation of pitch, elimination of hard glottic attacks • PPI, limit intake alcohol, smoking, caffeine, chocolate (all stimulate acid) • If resistant consider botox therapy (to decrease forceful adduction of arytenoids).

3.24 PARAPHARYNGEAL SPACE ABSCESS

CLINICAL PHOTOGRAPH	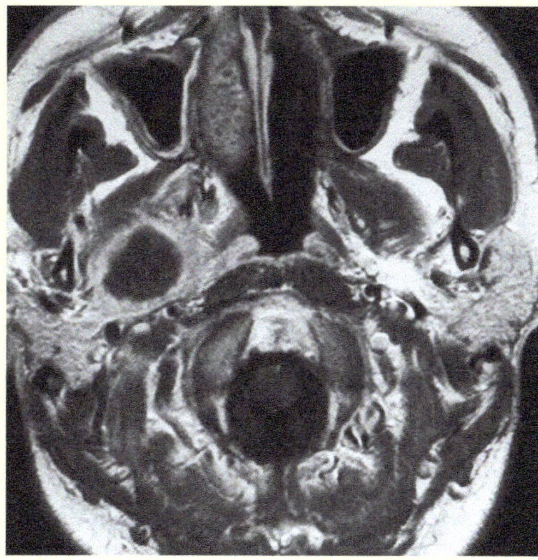

Introductory question	Answer
Describe the scan above.	• Axial T1 weighted MRI without contrast in the region of the suprahyoid neck (through Parapharyngeal space) • The most strike abnormality is ring enhancing lesion with central low intensity signal in the right parapharyngeal space

	• The most likely diagnosis is a parapharyngeal abscess (DD branchial cyst).
Competency question(s)	**Answer**
What signs and symptoms may be present?	• Trismus, Parotid oedema, Dysphagia, Retromandibular neck, mass, medial dispalcement of tonsil
What is the source of infection in such an abscess?	• Tonsil, Dental (3rd molar), Pharynx, Petrous temporal bone, Parotid, lymph node
How would you access the parapharyngeal space to drain this abscess?	• From the neck: the lateral aspect of the parapharyngeal space is bordered by the fascia of the posterior belly of the digastric muscle. Therefore cervical access for abscess drainage involves identifying and sectioning of the digastric muscle.
What are the boundaries of the parapharyngeal space?	• Superior - base of skull • Inferior - hyoid bone • Anterior - pterygomandibular raphe • Posterior – Fascia of tensor veli palatini • Medial - superior constrictor • Lateral - digastric muscle, Parotid,

	mandible, lat pterygoid
Advanced question(s)	**Answer**
What are the potential complications of a parapharyngeal abscess?	• Septic thrombosis • Carotid blowout • Cranial nerve involvement (horners, X, XII) • Mediastinitis • Pyopneumonithis • purulent pericarditis • bronchial erosion • aspiration pneumonia

3.25 GOITRE

CLINICAL PHOTOGRAPH	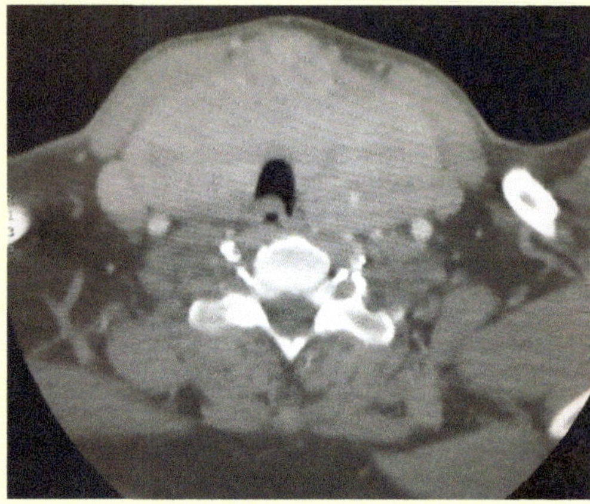

Introductory question	Answer
What is the abnormality shown in the image	• This is an axial CT scan through the neck at the level of the trachea showing a huge goitre • At the level shown there is no compromise to the tracheal airway.
Competency question(s)	**Answer**
What are the	Goitre aetiology may be divided into

causes a goitre?	subgroups as shown below: • *Physiological:* Puberty, increased metabolic demand pregnancy • *Autoimmune:* Graves' disease, Hashimoto's thyroiditis • *Thyroiditis:* Subacute granulomatous/de Quervain's, subacute lymphocytic, silent Riedel's thyroiditis, acute infective (transient) • *Granulomatous diseases:* Sarcoidosis, tuberculosis, Iodine deficiency, Idiopathic
During thyroidectomy how would you find the recurrent laryngeal nerve and the superior laryngeal nerve	• The recurrent laryngeal nerve is located in Beahr's triangle, which is formed by (1) the common carotid artery, (2) trachea and (3) inferior thyroid artery • The superior laryngeal nerve is found in Joll's triangle, which is formed by (1) the midline, (2) superior thyroid pedicle and (3) strap muscle.

Advanced question(s)	Answer
Tell me about the embryology of the thyroid gland.	• The thyroid is the 1st endocrine gland to develop • At 24th day gestation there is proliferation of *endodermal* epithelial cells on *median surface of pharyngeal floor* Between Tuberulum Impar (ant) and copula (post), known as foramen caecum • Thyroid precursor (thyroid primordium) starts as thickening and develops into thryoid diverticulum. Initially hollow, later solidifies and becomes bilobed.

3.26 NASOLABIAL CYST

CLINICAL IMAGE	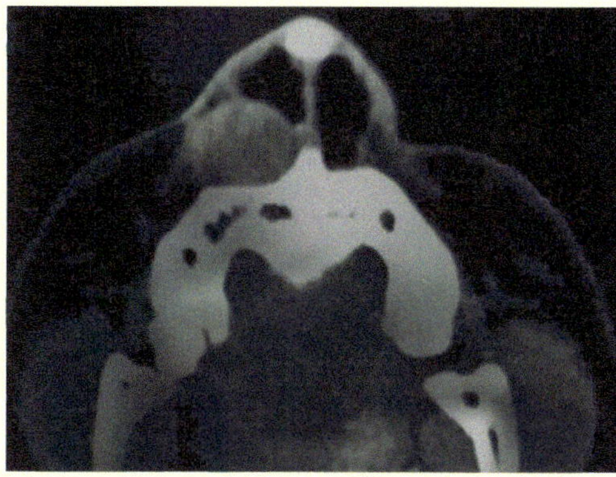

Introductory question	Answer
What is the abnormality in this CT scan?	• Axial CT soft tissue window image showing a lesion consistent with a nasolabial cyst (also known as a Klestadt's cyst, Non-odontogenic cyst, epithelial inclusion cyst, fissural cyst). • Less typical differentials include a neoplastic lesion (minor salivary gland tumour); skin appendage lesion, developmental abnormalities, odontogenic lesion.

Competency question(s)	Answer
What are the typical features of a nasolabial cyst? How would you treat this problem?	• Generally asymptomatic swelling under alar nasi,unilat nasal blockage; painful only if infected • Surgery via a sublabial approach is gold standard
Advanced question(s)	**Answer**
What is the aetiopathogenesis?	• Thought to arise from entrapped nasolacrimal tissue or entrapped nasolabial tissue (hence fissural cyst)

4.27 FREY'S SYNDROME AND BOTOX

CLINICAL PHOTOGRAPHS	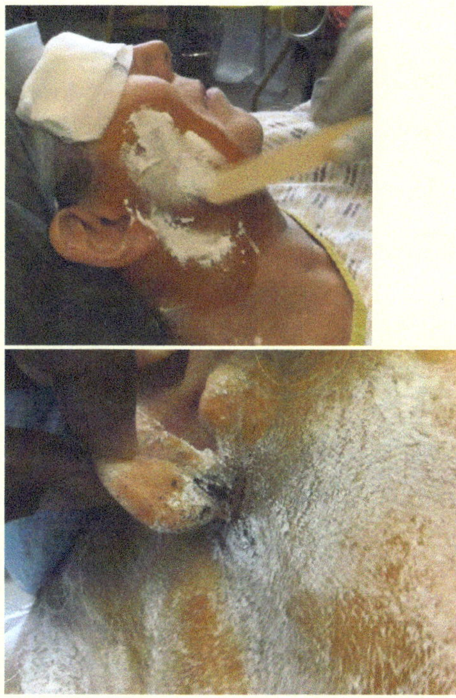

Introductory question	Answer
The patient is awake and asked	• Starch-iodine test for Frey's syndrome • There is a small positive reaction near the

to eat a few grapes after the white material is applied. What test is shown in the diagram?	right ear lobe suggestive of gustatory sweating.
Competency question(s)	**Answer**
What is Frey's syndrome?	• Frey's syndrome is also known as 'Gustatory sweating' and is related to parotid surgery or injury. • During surgery, parasympathetic secretomotor fibres innervate the parotid gland may be transected. The fibres regenerate in the skin where they assume control of sweat gland activity because of the common neurotransmitter acetylcholine. This inappropriate innervation results in facial sweating in response to salivatory stimuli.
How is the condition treated?	• Aluminium based deodorant • Topical glycopyrrolate • Botox injection • Neuronectomy (Jacobson's nerve section in the middle ear)
Tell me about	• Botulinum toxin (Botox) injection is now

Botox therapy?	the gold standard treatment for Frey's syndrome. Botox is a protease exotoxin, which works by blocking the release of acetylcholine from the cholinergic nerve end plates leading to inactivity of the glands or muscle innervated.
Advanced question(s)	**Answer**
Do you know of any other non-cosmetic therapeutic use for Botox, apart from Frey's syndrome?	• Yes, Botox has a role in multiple non-cosmetic head and neck conditions pertaining to larynx (spasmodic dysphonia), mouth (drooling), oesophagus (achalasia), face (hemifacial spasm), autonomic nervous system (first bite syndrome), pain (migraine) and nose (rhinitis) *For an evidence-based review of the use of Botox in non-cosmetic head and neck conditions, see Persaud et al. JRSM short report 2013; Feb 4 (2):10).*

3.28 GIANT PLEXIFORM NEUROFIBROMA OF SCALP

CLINICAL PHOTOGRAPH	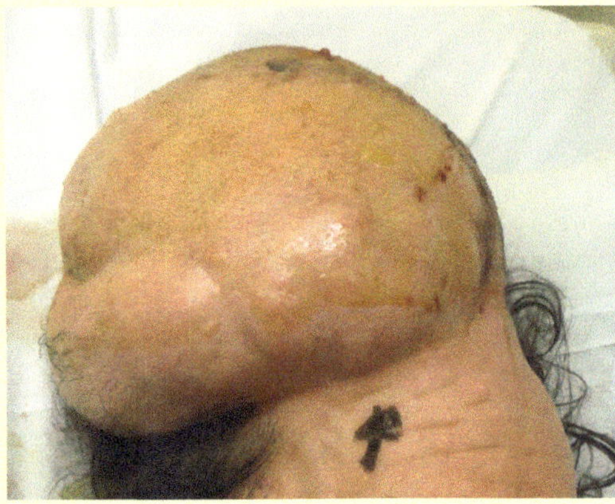

Introductory question	Answer
Describe what you see in the photograph	• Clinical photograph of a massive lesion on the head of a patient most likely to be benign or a benign tumour that has become malignant • Such lesion is consistent with neurofibroma, most likely plexiform neurofibroma (involving multiple peripheriphal nerves) rather than the dermal type which affects on one peripheral nerve.

Competency question(s)	Answer
Which condition is neurofibromas associated with?	• NF1 and NF2, both autosomal dominant conditions.
After having the lesion for 40 years the patient decides to have it removed. How would you perform the procedure?	• Joint case with a plastic surgeon to cover the resulting defect with a split skin graft **Surgical Steps** • The consented patient is anaesthesied and placed in a supine position with the lesion hanging over the northern edge of the operating table to allow easy access to the undersurface of the tumour. A circumferential incision line is drawn around the lesion and then Local anaesthesia is injected subcutaneously (zylocaine (1%) and adrenaline (1:100,000) . • The skin is incised with a scalpel initially and then monopolar diathermy is used. Haemostasis is achieved with diathermy and suture ties. Care is taken to locate and ligate branches of the superficial temporal arteries, which are the main blood supply to the tumour. • Dissection then proceeds in the plane between the periosteal layer and the capsule of the tumour. This results in bloodless dissection and separation of the tumour from the scalp.

	• The scalp is then prepared for the split-thickness skin graft by checking for any breach in the periosteal layer. Any denuded bony area is saucerised with a cutting bur to create a vascular bed so that the overlying split skin graft will remain viable. • Two separate large split-thickness skin grafts are harvested from the thigh and carefully prepared to cover the entire surgical defect on the scalp. • The skin grafts are carefully placed on the scalp, trimmed and secured with clips to the free skin edge; the two skin grafts were joined using 4.0 vicryl rapide . • Gelonet gauze is then applied over the split skin graft followed by copious amounts of chloramphenicol ointment . • Finally blue gauze, mefix adhesive dressing and a head hooded cap are added sequentially to further enhance the pressure dressing over the split-thickness skin graft.
Advanced question(s)	**Answer**
Do plexiform neurofibromas have malignant potential?	• Yes • Yes, a parotid tumour weighting 2.5kg (reported in ENTNews from Doncaster ENT Team)

The weight of the resected plexiform neurofibroma was exactly 3.4576 Kgs. Do you know the weight of the largest head and neck lesion previously resected in the UK? 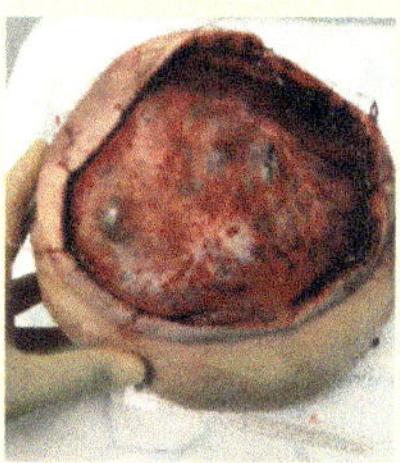 RESECTED SPECIMEN 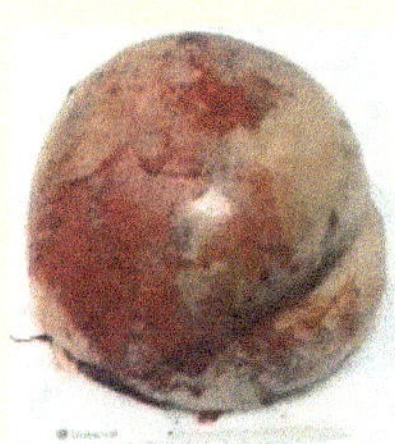	

CHAPTER 4

OTOLOGY and NEUROTOLOGY

4.1 ACUTE OTITIS EXTERNA

SCENARIO **(no clinical photograph)**	You are asked to see an 82 year old man with a 1 month history of an intermittently painful discharging right ear. The pain has recently become more persistent.

Introductory question	Answer
What is your differential diagnosis?	• Simple Otitis Externa (OE) • CSOM with perforation • Cholesteatoma • Necrotising Otitis Externa • Malignancy
Competency question(s)	**Answer**
How would you	• **History** –Essential to identify if there is a history of diabetes and treatment

proceed?	compliance; water exposure and cotton bud use; previous ear disease or surgery. • **Examination** – Careful otomicroscopy with microsuction plus take a swab for culture. • **Investigations –** Swab and Pure Tone Audiogram (PTA) initially. Consider high resolution CT (HRCT) temporal bones if suspicious of Necrotising OE (NOE). • **Treatment** – Meticulous aural toilet with regular microsuction is the mainstay of treatment. Topical antibiotic drops such as Ciprofloxacin, Sofradex or Gentisone is the primary treatment, guided by culture sensitivities. Oral or IV antibiotics are reserved for cases of NOE.
What is Necrotising Otitis Externa (NOE)?	• NOE is skull base osteitis secondary to uncontrolled otitis externa usually caused by pseudomonas infection. Typically in the elderly, diabetic or immunocompromised patient. A high level of suspicion is required for prompt diagnosis and treatment to avoid complications such as cranial nerve involvement. It is associated with a mortality of up to 50%.
How can it be further investigated and treated?	• A HRCT temporal bones looking for bony erosion or skull base involvement is the investigation of choice. Any suspicion of skull base osteomyelitis can be further investigated with a Gallium or Nuclear

	medicine white cell scan. HBA1C can delineate poor diabetic control. • Long term, high dose IV antibiotics are required, plus very regular aural toilet. Meticulous diabetic control is essential. • Surgical debridement of necrotic bone may be indicated, but is not routine. • Hyperbaric Oxygen treatment may have a role, and is currently undergoing trials.
Advanced question(s)	**Answer**
What are the constituents Locorten Vioform and is it safe to use when there is a perforation of the tympanic membrane?	• **Locorten-Vioform** = Flumetasone 0.02%, Clioquinol 1%. • Like ciprofloxacin ear drops, Locorten vioform is safe to use if there is a perforation in the tympanic membrane.
Do you know the constituents of any other ear drops?	• **Gentisone HC** = Hydrocortisone 1%, Gentamicin 0.3%. • **Otomize** = Dexamethasone 0.1%, Neomycin 3250 units/mL, Acetic acid 2%. • **Sofradex** = Dexamethasone 0.05%, Framycetin 0.5%, Gramicidin 0.005%

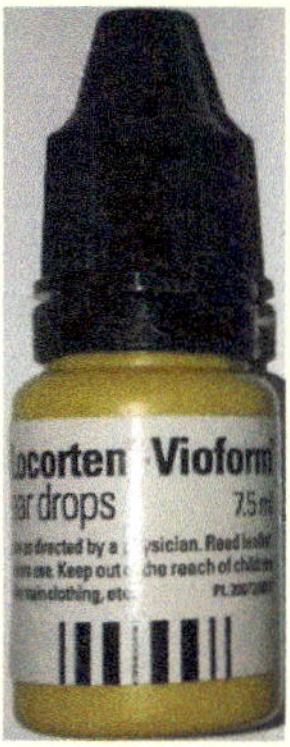Vioform	

4.2 EXOSTOSES AND OSTEOMAS

SCENARIO **(followed by a photograph)**	A 35 year old man presents with history of recurrent episodes of bilateral otitis externa. He works as a gardener and enjoys rowing and swimming. He is otherwise fit and well.

Introductory question	Answer
What are the causes of recurrent otitis externa?	• Water exposure • Cotton bud use • Foreign body • Exostoses • Skin conditions affecting the canal or meatus i.e. eczema, psoriasis • immunosuppression
Competency question(s)	**Answer**
This is what you see on otoscopy. What is this and how can it be managed?	• These are typical of ear canal exostoses. It occurs in patients who are regularly exposed to cold water and wind. This patient's outdoor occupation and hobbies put him at risk. • The exostoses are benign bony

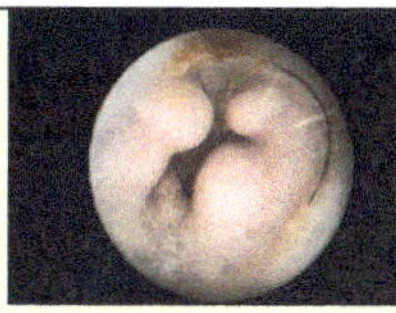	outgrowths of the tympanic ring. They occlude the canal and may lead to trapped wax and water becoming infected. In extreme cases they can even lead to conductive hearing loss. • Management includes advising ear protection from water and wind in mild cases, to surgical excision in extreme cases. The exostoses may be removed by drill or gauge, with careful preservation of the canal skin. • Risks to TMJ and facial nerve so pre-op CT important.
What are the differences between exostoses and osteoma?	• Exostoses occur medially, along the tympanic ring and are often bilateral. They are benign sessile bony outgrowths of cortical bone. • Osteomata occur at the bony-cartilagenous junction along suture lines and are usually unilateral. They are true neoplasms consisting of cancellous bone.
Advanced question(s)	**Answer**
Can osteomata of the ear canal be genetic?	• Yes. Gardner's syndrome, or familial colorectal polyposis is an autosomal dominant condition associated with formation of skull osteomata and is a genetic cause of ear canal osteoma. Patients may also present with multiple sebaceous cysts, fibromas and thyroid cancer. It is caused by a mutation in the APC gene on Chromosome 5q21.

4.3 PERFORATION OF TYMPANIC MEMBRANE

CLINICAL PHOTOGRAPH	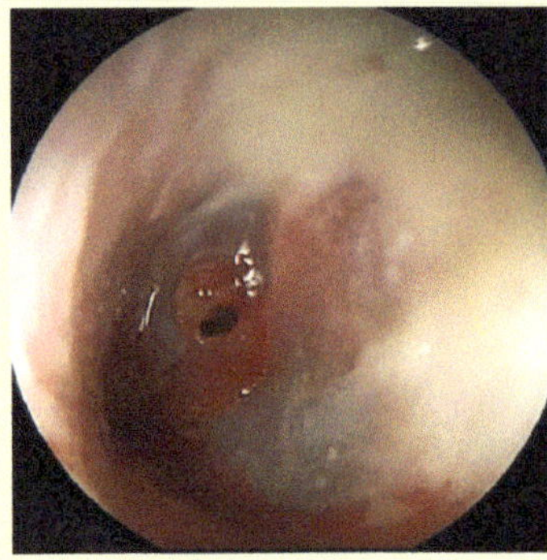

Introductory question	Answer
Describe the clinical photograph.	This is an endoscopic photograph of a left tympanic membrane with an anterior inferior central perforation with creamy discharge (pus) and blood in the deep ear canal.
Competency question(s)	**Answer**
What are the issues related to this condition and how would you manage them?	• The main issue is the increased risk of recurrent infection and discharge. • Recurrent discharge can be socially embarrassing and problematic. • Mainstay of treatment is protecting the ear from water to reduce the risk of

	infection. • Water precautions involve avid use of ear plugs or cotton wool with Vaseline and avoiding direct water contact to the ear. • It may be asymptomatic, in which case nothing other than water precautions are required.
Advanced question(s)	**Answer**
In problematic cases, how can this be treated?	• Careful discussion with the patient should involve the options of conservative versus surgical management in order to facilitate an informed choice. • Recurrent infection can lead to fibrosis and fixation of the ossicles resulting in a conductive hearing loss and sensorineural hearing loss can occur long term, secondary to ototoxic toxins secreted from the infecting organisms. • The risks and complications of Myringoplasty surgery should be discussed, including hearing loss, taste disturbance, graft failure, bleeding and infection. • This clinical picture may well represent a complication of grommet insertion, in view of the position of the perforation. In this case, myringoplasty may be complicated by recurrence of effusion, and this should be addressed.

4.4 TYMPANIC MEMBRANE RETRACTION

SCENARIO **(clinical photograph)**	A 28 year old man presents with hearing loss. There is no pain. He had a history of grommet insertion as a child but is otherwise fit and well. A pure tone audiogram reveals conductive hearing loss with an air-bone gap of 30dBHL on the left. Tympanometry reveals a "C-type" trace in the left ear. 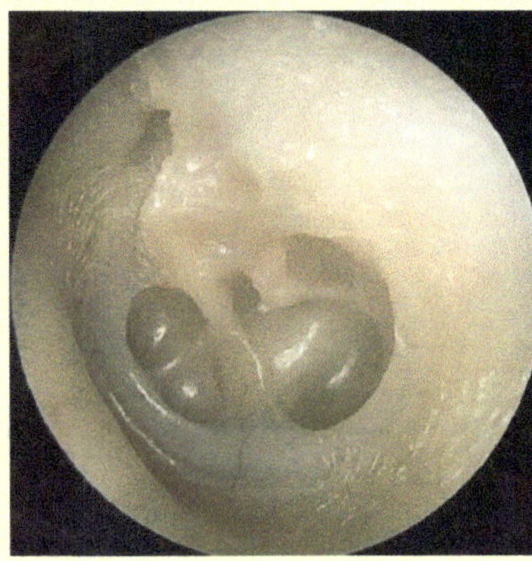

Introductory question	Answer
Describe this image?	• This is a clinical otoscopic photograph of a left tympanic membrane with retractions of both the *pars tensa* and *pars flaccida*. The incudostapedial joint is

	clearly visible.

Competency question(s)	Answer
How would you grade this?	• Retractions of the tympanic membrane are graded accordingly with the Sade system for *pars tensa* retractions and the Tos classification for *pars flaccida* retractions. • ***Sade Classification:*** Stage 1 – stretched annulus with a mild retraction Stage 2 – Retraction onto incudostapedial joint Stage 3 – Retraction onto promontory (lifts on valsalva) Stage 4 – Adherent to promontory
What is the risk of a retraction pocket?	• ***Tos Classification:*** Grade 1 – **d**imple or mild retraction Grade 2 – **d**raping over neck of malleus Grade 3 – **d**istruction of scutum Grade 4 – **d**eep retraction with keratin (synonymous with cholesteatoma)
How would you manage this?	• Progression with erosion of ossicles and development of cholesteatoma. • This is controversial and it is very

	important to know the status of the other ear. • The mainstay is close observation, scrupulous cleaning when necessary and protection from water/moisture to avoid infection. • Debris and keratin build up must be removed regularly to prevent the development of cholesteatoma. • Improve middle ear ventilation to prevent progression. - Regular valsalva manoeuvres - Use of inflation devices such as Otovent balloon. - Nasal treatment if signs of rhinitis/postnasal space oedema - Grommet insertion in selected patients. If symptomatic with recurrent infection/discharge consider reinforcement Tympanoplasty.
Advanced question(s)	**Answer**
Describe the embryology and structure of the tympanic membrane.	• There are 3 layers to the tympanic membrane held on a fibrous annulus attached to the tympanic ring of the temporal bone. • The outer layer is the epidermal squamous layer (skin). It is formed, along with the external auditory canal, from

	ectoderm of the first branchial cleft. • The middle fibrous lamina propria layer is formed from mesoderm. Its structure is of concentric circles of type II collagen with radial strands adding reinforcement. On either side of this stiff layer are loose-connective tissue layers containing nerve fibres and a vascular plexus. • The inner layer is mucosal and is formed, along with the mucosa of the middle ear, from the endoderm of the first branchial pouch. • The pars flaccida has some fibrous tissue but it is not as well organised as the layer in the pars tensa and this results in a lack of rigidity.

4.5 CHOLESTEATOMA OF THE MIDDLE EAR

CLINICAL PHOTOGRAPH	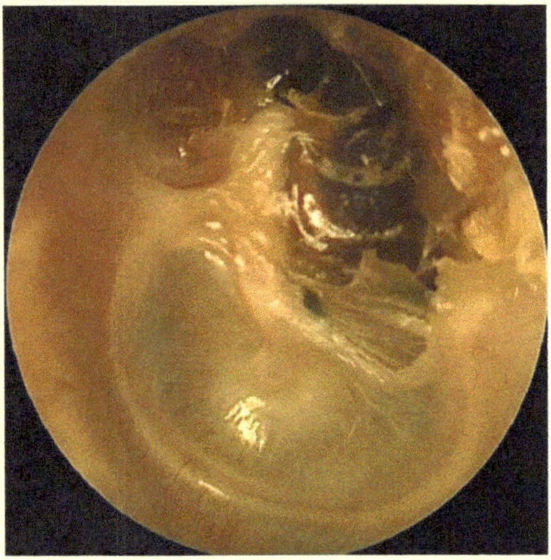

Introductory question	Answer
Describe the photograph?	• This is a clinical otoscopic photograph of a left tympanic membrane with a frank attic cholesteatoma. (The dark discolouration is due to oxidised keratin).
Competency question(s)	**Answer**
What is cholesteatoma	• Cholesteatoma is a collection of KERATINISING squamous epithelium

and how is it caused?	leading to bone and soft tissue erosion as well as infection. It is most commonly found in the middle ear cleft, but can occur elsewhere such as the external ear canal. • There are 4 general types: - Primary acquired = occurs in a retraction pocket secondary to negative middle ear pressure. - Hyperplasia and migration following chronic inflammation - Secondary acquired = migration of epithelial cells through a perforation, or implanted via trauma or iatrogenically. - Congenital = embryonic epithelial rests in the middle ear with an intact tympanic membrane (also know as epidermoid formation or Michael's body – after the Otopathologist Leslie Michael who re-discovered it).
What are the issues related to this condition?	• Cholesteatoma is associated with chronic infection and discharge. • If left untreated, a cholesteatoma will slowly progress. This occurs through a combination of persistent low middle ear pressure, further migration of epithelial cells into the cholesteatoma, proliferation and the release of osteolytic enzymes. • Progressive expansion and infection of the cholesteatoma can lead to

	complications. These are subdivided into otological complications, extra and intracranial complications. • Otologic (Intra-temporal) complications; - Destruction of the ossicular chain - Hearing loss (conductive and sensorineural) - Perilymph fistula (Vertigo) - Facial nerve damage (Palsy) - Acute mastoiditis - Petrositis (Gradenigo syndrome) • Extra-cranial complications - External abcesses - Subperiosteal mastoid abscess - Bezold Abscess (sternomastoid) - Citelli Abscess (digastric) - Lucs Abscess (temporalis) • Intra-cranial Complications - Meningitis - Extradural, Subdural abscesses - Intracerebral abscess - Cerebritis/encephalitis

	- Lateral/sigmoid sinus thrombosis - Hydrocephalus
Advanced question(s)	**Answer**
What do you see in this CT scan? 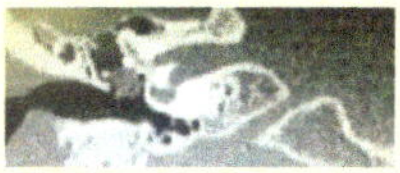	Coronal CT showing a small lesion in the middle ear. I may represent a cholesteatoma, granulation tissue or glomus tympanicum
Describe this photograph 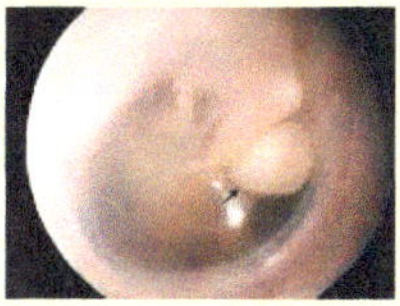	Otoscopic view of the right tympanic membrane should an intact drum with a pearly white lesion in the anterior superior quadrant. This is likely to represent a congenital cholesteatoma as it is the typical position to find such a lesion.
What do understand by DWI?	DWI is Diffusion Weighted Imaging. This refers to Diffusion-weighted echo-planar Magnetic Resonance Imaging. This can be used as a pre-operative scanning modality or as an alternative to second look in combined approach tympanoplasty patients. It can distinguish between inflammatory tissue and cholesteatoma, where other imaging modalities cannot.

4.6 OTOSCLEROSIS

SCENARIO (followed by an audiogram)	GP referral: A 40 year old woman is referred to the ENT clinic with a left sided hearing loss. Examination confirms the tympanic membranes to be normal in appearance, whilst audiometry demonstrates a mixed pattern bilateral loss, worse on the left, with the predominant component being conductive.

Introductory question	Answer
What other questions would you ask in the history to further determine the possible cause of the conductive hearing loss?	**History:** Length of history (any childhood history); history of previous ear infections; previous ear surgery; history of trauma to the ear (direct / barotrauma); any noise exposure history; family history of ear problems; did hearing get worse during any previous pregnancy; tinnitus, balance disturbance.

Competency question(s)	Answer
Look at the audiogram. Considering this and the clinical history, what is the likely diagnosis? 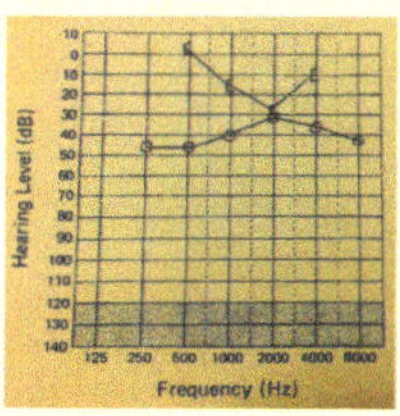	• The audiogram shows a conductive hearing in the right ear with a Cahart's notch. In the presence of a type A tympanogram, the most likely diagnosis would be otosclerosis.
How would you manage the patient?	• **Management** – history/examination. ***Investigations*** – stapedial reflexes, speech audiogram, high resolution CT scan temporal bones looking at stapes footplate. ***Treatment*** – conservative with monitoring, hearing aid, stapedectomy, fluoride treatment (Not currently recommended. Fluoride incorporates into hydroxyapatite. Treatment monitored by absence of Schwartze's (Flamingo blush) sign if present and serial audiometry. Discuss negatives – stomach ulceration, arthritis, osteopenia).
• How do you classify	• Footplate classification (Ludman,

variations in the footplate and what is the surgical significance of this?	originally postulated by Belluci): Type I - stapes minimally fixed in oval window Type 2 - thin footplate, resists perforation more than I Type 3 - thick footplate Type 4 - fixed to oval window, can only be perforated by drilling. Relevance relates to degree of ease of stapedotomy and possibility of floating stapes footplate.
Advanced question(s)	**Answer**
What are the pre-operative and intra-operative contraindications to stapedectomy?	• Contraindications to stapedectomy: - **Preoperative**: only hearing ear; predominant cochlear component or minimal air bone gap; tinnitus or vertigo as predominant symptoms; active foci as judged by positive Schwartz sign; minimal likelihood of significant improvement in hearing impairment as judged by Glasgow Benefit Plot. - **Intraoperative**: Incorrect diagnosis; floating footplate (could try to elevate but dangerous as risk of permanent SNHL); low stapedial artery crossing footplate; perilymph gusher; overhanging facial nerve Severe dizziness post stapedectomy: Clinical assessment first (is it fluctuant),

	examination, audiometry, CT scan if persists, to check position of piston. May not be related to stapedectomy. If hearing deficit or fluctuant consider re-exploration.

4.7 MENIERE'S DISEASE

SCENARIO (no clinical photograph)	You have been referred a 45 year old lady with episodic dizziness. She has also developed right sided tinnitus. On further questioning she states that she has been having difficulty using the telephone with her right ear recently. She has a history of migraine. She is otherwise fit and well with no regular medication.

Introductory question	Answer
What is your differential diagnosis?	• Right-sided Meniere's disease. • Right Vestibulopathy. • Vestibular Neuronitis. • Vestibular Migraine.
Competency question(s)	**Answer**
How would you proceed?	• **History** – The most important questions are; - Is this Vertigo? - What is the duration of the Vertigo? - Are there any associated symptoms? • Vertigo is a hallucination of movement

	and is the cardinal symptom of vestibular dysfunction. Other non-specific dizziness symptoms point to a cardiac or neurological cause. • The duration of the vertigo is key; - Secs to mins = likely Benign Paroxysmal Positional Vertigo (BPPV). - Hours = likely Meniere's, Migraine or Vestibulopathy - Days = Vestibular Neuronitis. - Continuous = central or psychogenic • Associated hearing loss, increase in tinnitus intensity and/or an aural fullness during attack suggests Meniere's. Headache associated with the attack suggests vestibular migraine, as does aura or parasymathetic symptoms. There is a significant overlap with Meniere's and Migraine with up to 40% of patients having both conditions simultaneously. • **Examination** – Otoscopy for disease, Cranial nerve examination in central causes, Romberg and Unterberger tests looking for proprioceptive and peripheral vestibular signs, and Dix-Hallpike test for BPPV. Hamalgi Head-thrust test to elicit vestibulo-occular reflex (VOR) abnormalities. Look carefully for spontaneous and provoked nystagmus. Examination often normal unless there are concurrent symptoms.
How would you treat a diagnosis of Meniere's	

disease?	• **Investigations –**Hearing testing with tuning fork tests and pure tone audiogram. MRI of Internal Acoustic Meati looking for vestibular schwannoma indicated by unilateral hearing loss and tinnitus. In equivocal cases or suspected vestibulopathy, Video or Electronystagmography (VNG, ENG) and Caloric testing. • A stepwise approach is used. • Simple lifestyle and dietary changes help in most cases. Reducing Salt, caffeine and alcohol can help in a large number of cases. • Drug therapy with Betahistine and/or Bendroflumethazide is used effectively in many patients. Prochlorperazine can be used when required for symptomatic relief during the vertigo. • For those patients uncontrolled with the above, intratympanic steroid has been shown to provide some improvement. • Endolymphatic sac decompression surgery is effective in some. • Ultimately, for those resistant or debilitating cases, labyrinthectomy is used. This can be either chemical via intratympanic gentamycin or surgical. • When Meniere's is stable, vestibular rehabilitation is very useful.

Advanced question(s)	Answer
Do you know of any other tests for Meniere's disease?	• Vestibular-Evoked Myogenic Potentials (VEMPs) and Electrocochleography (ECochG)
Can you explain what these are and draw an ECochG trace?	• VEMP is a test whereby an auditory stimulation (95bD click) passes via the saccule and inferior vestibular nerve (IVN) to the vestibular nucleus. A reflex arc then stimulates the ipsilateral sternocleidomastoid (SCM) muscle via the vestibulospinal tract. This, detected by an action potential in the SCM is delayed in Meniere's Disease, along with any IVN lesion such as vestibular schwannoma, or saccular dysfunction. In superior semicircular canal dehiscence the potential is increased. • ECochG is the recording of electrical potentials in the auditory nerve and cochlea in response to auditory clicks via air conduction. A probe is placed on or near the tympanic membrane with a reference electrode on the mastoid and forehead. It can detect Endolymphatic hydrops in Meniere's by an increase in the summation potential/Compound Action Potential ratio.

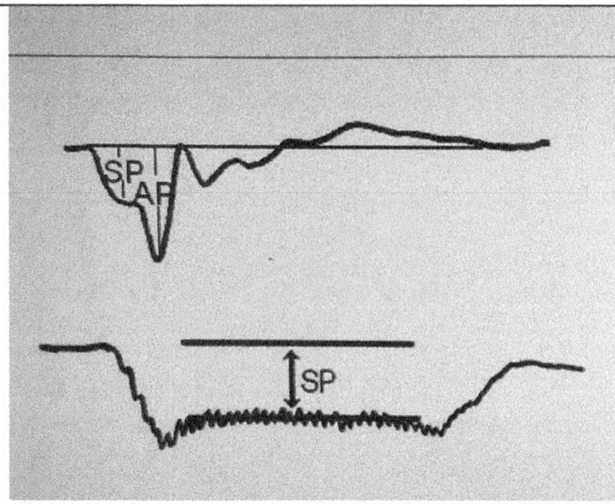

It is essentially an 'ECG' of inner ear function (Outer Hair Cells (OHCs), Basilar membrane & Vestibulocochlear nerve (CN8))

Abnormal in hydrops.

Transtympanic TT vs extratympanic ET active electode (TT response 10 times larger)

Click stimulus (traditional) but short tone bursts give better results; 1kHz tone burst provides the best indication of hydrops.

The three section of the ECochG are:

1. Cochlear microphonics - reflects OHCs function.
2. Summation Potential (SP) - basilar membrane 'set point'.
3. Action Potential (AP) - reflects CN8.

The ratio of amplitude of SP/AP is used for measurement in disease;

Generally abnormal if ratio >40% (range 34-47%) (published studies).

4.8 BENIGN PAROXSYMAL POSITIONAL VERTIGO

CLINICAL PHOTOGRAPH	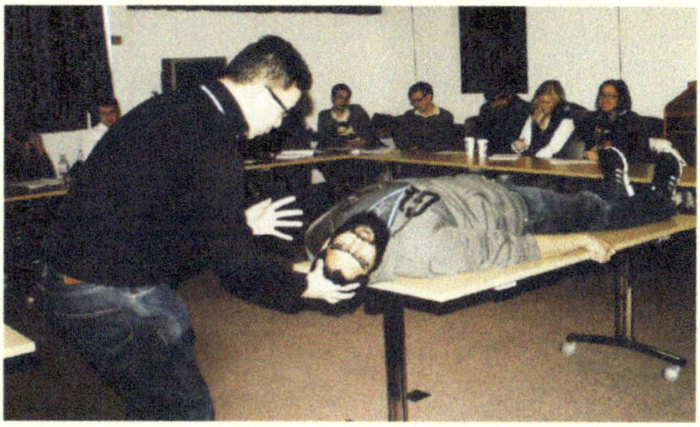

Introductory question	Answer
Describe what is being done in the photograph.	This is a clinical photograph of a patient undergoing a particle repositioning manoeuvre such as Epley.
Competency question(s)	**Answer**
What is Dix-Hallpike test?	• The Dix-Hallpike test is diagnostic of Benign Positional Paroxysmal Vertigo (BPPV). There is usually a short latency of around 2-10 secs after which a positive test shows a torsional nystagmus, usually towards the test ear, or the floor (Geotropic) (or other nystagmus types in rare cases – see below)

What is the pathophysiology of BPPV?	• BPPV is the most common peripheral vestibular condition presenting in balance clinics. • It is characterised by short-lived episodes of vertigo lasting seconds to minutes at a time and provoked by changes in head position. The most common provoking positions are lying down and turning in bed, looking up and bending down. • In pure BPPV there are no other otological symptoms such as hearing loss or tinnitus, although they may co-exist. • It often occurs spontaneously, but other aetiological factors include head injury, post-viral (vestibular neuronitis), post-surgical. • It is often self-limiting. • There are two theories of pathophysiology. - Canalithiasis. Dislodged otoconia from the saccule/utricle float freely in the endolymph of the semicircular canal. The inertial effect of their movement in the fluid causes cupula displacement and short-lived vertigo which resolves when the otoconia come to rest. - Cupulolithiasis. Loose otoconia become adherent to the cupula causing stimulation due to gravity on movement. Treatment of BPPV following a positive Dix-Hallpike test is with a particle repositioning

	manoeuvre such as the Epley.
Advanced question(s)	**Answer**
Are you aware of the different types of BPPV? How do these types differ clinically?	• Yes, there are 3 types. The most common, accounting for up to 90% is Posterior canal BPPV. Lateral, or Horizontal BPPV accounts for over 8% and Superior canal BPPV is extremely rare, accounting for less than 1% of cases. • Lateral canal BPPV tends to present with more severe and prolonged symptoms. • Lateral canal BPPV elicits a horizontal nystagmus on Dix-Hallpike test rather than a torsional nystagmus. It may be Geotropic (75%) or Ageotropic (25%). The supine roll test (patient supine with head rolled to side) is an alternative to Dix-Hallpike for this. Treatment requires a Barbecue 360° roll manoeuvre. • Superior canal BPPV is very rare due to the position of the canal. • Superior canal BPPV exhibits a downbeating nystagmus on Dix-Hallpike testing without a torsional element. • All episodes of downbeating nystagmus should be investigated as a central cause for this is more common than a superior

	canal BPPV.
Is there a surgical treatment for BPPV?	• Yes. Semicircular canal occlusion can be performed in intractable or disabling cases. It involves access to the canals via a cortical Mastoidectomy approach and plugging the affected canal with bone pate, muscle and fascia.

4.9 TEMPORAL BONE FRACTURE

SCENARIO **(no clinical photograph)**	A 35 year old man presents in the Emergency Department (ED) having fallen from his bicycle. He lost consciousness for 5 minutes. ED have cleared him from a head injury point of view, but have referred him as he is complaining of bleeding and hearing loss in his left ear.

Introductory question	**Answer**
What is your differential diagnosis?	There has clearly been some ear trauma here, but it is important to determine if it is simple blunt trauma or a bony fracture.
Competency question(s)	**Answer**
How can you determine the difference?	• Hearing loss may be conductive secondary to haemotympanum or ossicular disruption, or sensorineural secondary cochlea injury in fracture. • Bleeding may be caused by a traumatic perforation or a fracture that passes into the ear canal. • Careful examination should include facial nerve assessment and looking for signs

	such as nystagmus and CSF leak. • Audiogram must be performed if there is a history of hearing loss or it is identified by tuning fork tests. • Tympanogram is contraindicated as it may provoke a pneumocephalus. • A CT scan should be performed if fracture is suspected. Angiogram if carotid injury is suspected, or where the fracture involves the foramen lacerum.
This is the CT scan. What does it show? 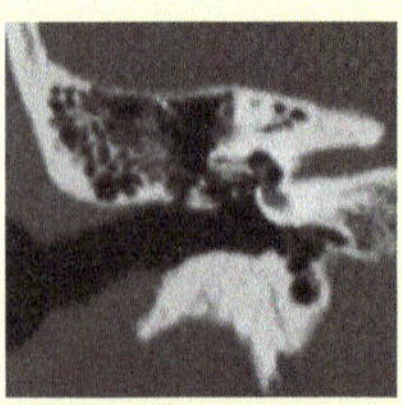	This image shows a longitudinal fracture as well as a transverse fracture of the petrous temporal bone with a pneumolabyrinth. This patient will have an irreversible dead ear.
Advanced question(s)	**Answer**
What are the differences between longitudinal and transverse fractures?	• Longitudinal are more common than transverse fractures by 75% to 25%. They tend to occur by a lateral blow whereas transverse fractures are caused by fronto-occipital force. • Longitudinal fractures rarely cause cochlea injury whereas a transverse fracture is associated with cochlea and

	IAC injury. • Longitudinal is associated with conductive hearing loss due to haemotympanum or ossicular discontinuity. Transverse is associated with sensorineural loss due to cochlea or IAC injury. • Both types of fracture can result in haemotympanum, but longitudinal fractures are more often associated with laceration through the tympanic membrane and external canal fracture therefore bleeding from the ear. • Facial nerve injury is far more likely from transverse fractures. • Delayed nerve palsy may occur due to oedema and ischaemia of the nerve.
How else may temporal bone fracture be classified?	• Temporal bone fracture with or without immediate facial nerve palsy.
How can one determine if a clear fluid leak from the ear is CSF?	• The presence of Beta-2-transferrin which is ONLY found in CSF and endolymph.

4.10 NOISE-INDUCED HEARING LOSS

<table>
<tr>
<td>SCENARIO
(and audiogram)</td>
<td>You are asked to see a 32yrs-old who complains of a blocked ear following years of attending rock concerts. The pure tone audiogram reveals the following:

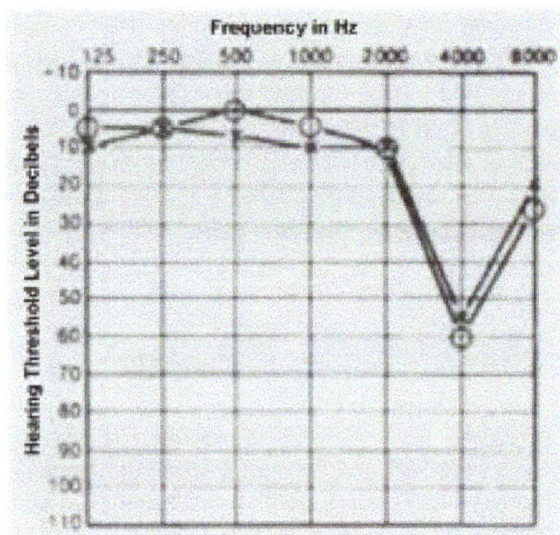

</td>
</tr>
</table>

Introductory question	Answer
Please describe what the PTA shows.	Normal Left and right air conduction thresholds with a 60dB dip at 4000Hz followed by a partial recover.

Competency question(s)	Answer
What is the likely diagnosis and how would you manage this patient?	• This pattern of SNHL with loss at 3-6KHz and recovery at 8KHz is in keeping with noise induced hearing loss. A formal diagnosis requires an awareness of noise exposure from other sources reference to age standardised normograms for hearing thresholds. • Management is largely preventative for future noise exposure with ear plugs (10-15dbl attenuation) and ear muffs (15-20dbl attenuation). • Co-existing tinnitus and hyperacusis may need to be managed with counselling if appropriate.
Advanced question(s)	**Answer**
What is the mechanism of noise induced hearing loss? How could you develop a strategy to treat this condition?	• Outer hair cells and then inner hair cell loss via apoptotic and necrotic mechanisms resulting from oxidative stress and excito-toxicity • Loss is potentiated by concomitant use of ototoxic medication or genetic predisposition. • 4KHz may be preferentially degraded as the resonant frequency of the Organ of Corti. If the patient presents early enough <72hrs empirical laboratory data suggest that there

	may be a role for drugs to prevent the production of free radicals and the calcium led apoptotic pathway via steroids and calcineurin antagonists.

4.11 NON-ORGANIC HEARING LOSS

SCENARIO (Audiograms)	GP referral: A 55 year old patient is referred to the ENT clinic from the direct access audiology service with an asymmetric hearing loss

Introductory question	Answer
• Look at the audiogram and describe the abnormalities . • 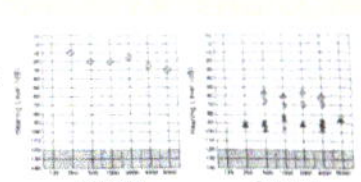	• The right ear shows unmasked air conduction thresholds which when averaged is just within the normal range. • Unmasked bone conduction is reduced to 60dBHL average. • The left ear shows a mixed hearing loss with masked bone conduction at around 70dBHL and masked air conduction at around 90dBHL.

Competency question(s)	Answer
What is the most likely diagnosis?	• Reduced unmasked BC raises the suspicion of a **non organic hearing loss**, as even in the presence of a hearing loss in one ear, unmasked BC thresholds should be heard in the contralateral (good) ear.

Advanced question(s)	Answer
Which other tests would you consider to confirm your suspicion that the hearing loss is non-organic? 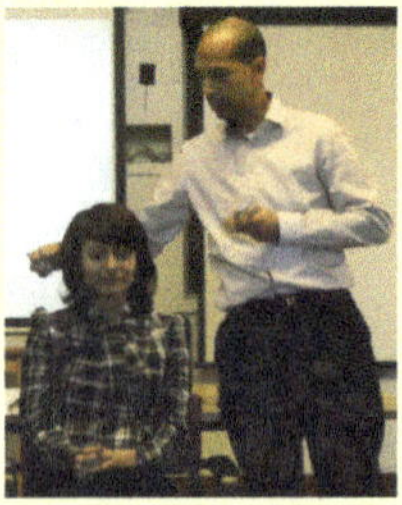 What test is being carried out here?	• **Subjective:** - Stengers tuning fork test: Based on the Stenger's phenomenon in which only the louder of two similar tones presented to both ears at the same time will be heard. - Chimani-Moos: the patient does not accept that they hear Weber's better in occluded ear; Lombards (raise voice level in response to noisy environment); delayed speech feedback test; • **Objective:** Maintenance of cochlea-auricular palpebral reflexes; ABRs, CERA (gold standard). • Also suspect if voice normal (only if bilateral non-organic), if gross discrepancy between pure tone and speech audiometry. • Stenger's test is been demonstrated.

Table 5.11a Tuning fork tests for sorting out the malingerer

TUNING FORK TESTS	DESCRIPTION
Stenger test (Stenger 1900)	• ***Principle*** – Sound presented in both ears will only be heard in the ear where the sound is louder

	• ***Test*** – 2 tuning forks of same frequency used – Eyes closed/blindfolded – 1st tuning fork to good ear at 15cm (heard), then removed – 2nd tuning fork to deaf ear at 5cm (not heard), not removed – Re-introduce 1st tuning fork to good ear at 15cm (heard if not a malingerer) • ***Malingerer Response*** – Denys hearing any sound as can only hear sound in feigned 'deaf' ear
Teal test	• ***Principle*** – Conductive hearing • ***Test*** – Vibrating tuning fork to mastoid of 'deaf' ear (heard) – Patient blind-folded and advised test to be repeated – Non-vibrating tuning fork to 'deaf' ear and simultaneously vibrating tuning fork near EAC of same ear (not heard if not a malingerer) • ***Malingerer Response*** – Will claim to hear sound as will assume through bone conduction when it is actually through air conduction

Chimani Moos test	• ***Principle*** – Variation of Weber test • ***Test*** – Tuning fork place on vertex – Heard in good ear – EAC occluded in good ear (heard in good ear still) • ***Malingerer Response*** – Deny hearing any sound at all

Table 5.11b Voice tests for sorting out the malingerer (by Julian Gaskin, FRCS (ORL-HNS).

VOICE TESTS	DESCRIPTION
Lombard	• ***Principle*** – Person will raise voice in speaking in noisy environment • ***Test*** – Patient asked to read text aloud without stopping – Noise introduced into good ear (i.e. Barany box) – Patient's voice will get louder • ***Malingerer Response*** – Will continue to read at even tone
Hummel double conservation test	• ***Principle*** – 2 different voices introduced into either ear will create confusion • ***Test*** – A question is asked into one ear and a different question asked into the other – If deaf in one ear there will be no confusion • ***Malingerer Response*** – Confusion or no response

Erhardt test (loud voice test)	• ***Principle*** – Occlusion of the EAC causes attenuation of 30dB • ***Test*** – Good ear is occluded with a finger – Sound projected into that ear – Normally, the patient will be able to hear the dampened sound • ***Malingerer Response*** – Denies hearing *any* sound at all, even when sound increased
Delayed speech feedback test	• ***Principle*** – Delayed sound introduced into the other ear will create confusion • ***Test*** – Patient asked to read text aloud without stopping – His voice is recorded and played back via headphones with 2ms delay into deaf ear • ***Malingerer Response*** – Confusion, change reading pattern (stammer, slow, raise voice)

4.12 DRUG-INDUCED HEARING LOSS

SCENARIO (followed by PTAs)	A 64 year old man with pulmonary tuberculosis (TB) had a relapse despite a four month course of high dose anti-tuberculous drugs. He was started on Amikacin, an aminoglycoside antibiotic which is used in multidrug-resistant TB. Two months into treatment, he complained of a mild deterioration in the hearing in his left ear. There are no other otological symptoms.

Introductory question	Answer
Describe this PTA 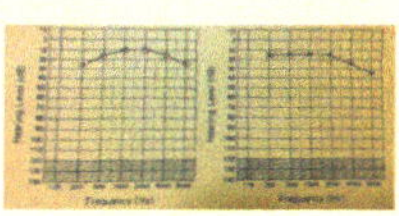	• This is a pure tone audiogram with the X-axis representing increasing frequency of pure tones and the Y-axis representing hearing level in Decibels (dB). • Only unmasked air conduction is recorded in the right ear (represented by an open circle) and left ear (represented by a cross). • It shows hearing, which on average is within normal limits, however, there is a slight difference between the two sides with a mild low-frequency loss in the right ear and a mild high-frequency loss in the left ear.

Competency question(s)	Answer
Describe this change in PTA 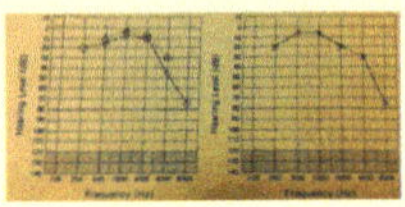	• This PTA records both air conduction in each ear and unmasked bone conduction in the right ear. • The traces recorded show a bilateral high-frequency sensorineural hearing loss.
What is the diagnosis?	• Given the history of the prolonged use of an aminoglycoside antibiotic, and the PTA, a diagnosis of drug-induced ototoxic hearing loss is most probable. Certain aminoglycosides such as Amikacin have narrow therapeutic windows and as such too high a dose can lead to ototoxicity. • Ototoxicity is defined as a greater than 10dB reduction in hearing at one or more frequency bilaterally. • It most commonly affects high frequencies initially, progressing to involve the lower frequencies.
How would you treat ototoxicity?	• Immediately stop the offending drug if the clinical condition permits. Consider alternative medication. In the vast majority of cases, once the ototoxic drug is withdrawn, the hearing will return to normal within a few days. However, in some cases there may be a permanent deficit.

	• It is important to exclude other causes of sensorineural hearing loss in these patients, and investigate accordingly. • Amplification may be required to improve the hearing. When profound or total loss occurs, cochlea implantation can be considered.
Advanced question(s)	**Answer**
What other drugs can cause ototoxicity and how does it occur?	• Ototoxicity is common with aminoglycoside antibiotics, along with other drugs such as macrolides, loop diuretics, salicylates, quinine, heavy metals and chemotherapeutic agents. • The drugs leach into the endolymph of the inner ear and cause direct damage to the outer hair cells initially and later the inner hair cells. Damage can also occur to the vestibular apparatus. • The hair cell damage is thought to occur as the result of free-radical damage from reactive oxygen species as a result of the drug action.

4.13 BONE ANCHORED HEARING AID (BAHA)

CLINICAL PHOTOGRAPH	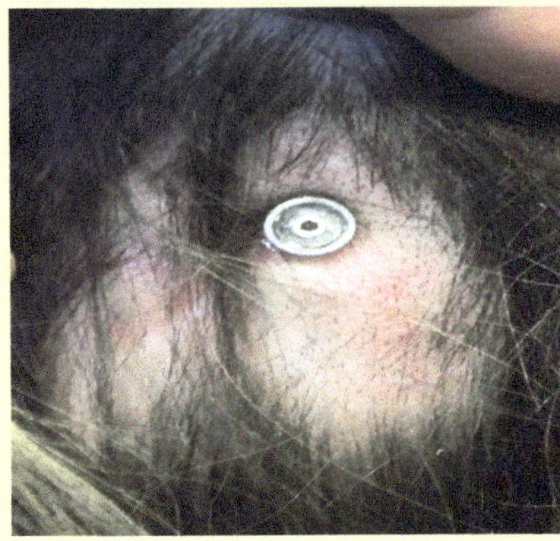

Introductory question	Answer
What is the name of device?	• Trans-cutaneous abutment for a bone anchored hearing aid (BAHA).
Competency question(s)	**Answer**
What are the main indications for this device?	**Two indications** • **Primary group**: patients unable to benefit from air conduction hearing aid due to: persistently discharging ear, canal stenosis, microtia. Best suited to conductive loss with adequate bone conduction thresholds. Processor power

	prescribed according to bone conduction thresholds (e.g. <35dBHL Divino, <45dBHL Intenso, <55dBHL Cordelle).
What are the main complications of the BAHA and how might they be overcome?	• **Secondary group** is patients with profound unilateral hearing loss with adequate contra-lateral bone conduction thresholds e.g. following vestibular schwannoma resection. The device reduces the head shadow effect, improves sound localisation and speech in noise discrimination. • NB Surgery in adults is typically performed as a single stage procedure with device loading 4 weeks post implantation. • Soft tissue overgrowth / local inflammation and peri-implant pain. • Historically they have been overcome by complete soft tissue reduction allowing skin to adhere to bone at the point of implant interface. • Recent advances include the development of longer abutments which do not require soft tissue reduction as well as abutments coated with osteoneogenic hydroxyapatite to encourage tissue adherence. • Skin punch implantation may also reduce the likelihood for local chronic pain due

	to sparing of occipital nerve branches during surgery.
Advanced question(s)	**Answer**
What are the different types of BAHA available and their BC thresholds?	• DIVINO < 35dBHL • INTENSO < 45dBHL • CORDELLE < 55dBHL • BODY WORN < 55 dBHL • Speech Discrimination < 60% in general
How does the saphano works?	• Implantable magnets used instead of a transcutaneous titanium screw.

4.14 COCHLEAR IMPLANT

CLINICAL PHOTOGRAPHS	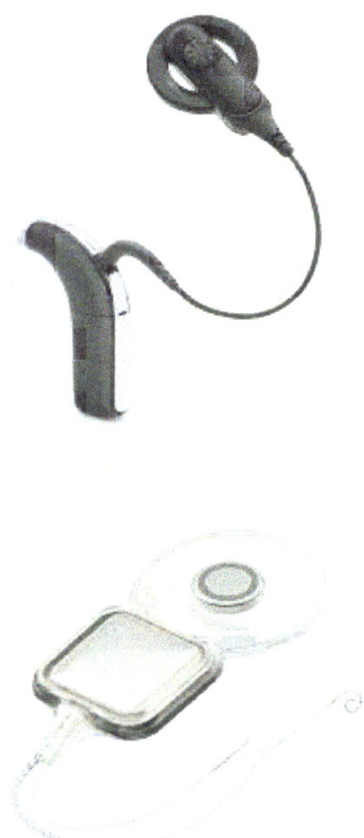

Introductory question	Answer
What is this device?	• Cochlear implant (CI) receiver and stimulator package.

Competency question(s)	Answer
Who are the traditional candidate groups for this device and what are their candidacy criteria?	• The traditional candidate groups are: 1. Pre-lingually deafened children who are offered simultaneous bilateral implants 2. Post-lingually deafened adults are offered unilateral implants unless visually impaired. • **Adult candidacy criteria** is bilateral severe to profound hearing loss (≥90dBHL at 2 and 4 KHz) who do not receive adequate benefit from acoustic hearing aids ***(<50% Bamford-Kowal-Bench sentence scores at 70dBSPL)*** • **Child candidacy criteria** is bilateral severe to profound hearing loss (≥90dBHL at 2 and 4 KHz) whose speech, language or listening skills have not developed or are not maintained at a level appropriate to developmental age and cognitive ability of the child. • Both groups should be assessed by CI MDT groups and have a 3month trial of acoustic hearing aids (unless contra-indicated or inappropriate) • Investigative work-up includes CT scan to exclude cochlear obliteration and MR scan to ensure the presence of an acoustic nerve in children.

Advanced question(s)	Answer
What is electro-acoustic stimulation and what is its role in cochlear implantation?	• It is the process of stimulating the cochlear with both electrical stimulation via the implant electrode and also by an acoustic hearing aid to the same device, in separate devices, or by a hybrid processor. • It is possible in patients with significant residual low frequency hearing with thresholds under 65dBHL at 250 and 500Hz. This residual capacity may be preserved by 'soft surgical techniques' including round window electrode insertion, topical corticosteroid and new electrode design. • Early studies suggest that patients obtain greater benefit in the speech in noise scenario and a greater appreciation for music.

4.15 CHRONIC OTITIS EXTERNA

SCENARIO **(no clinical photograph)**	GP referral: Please could you see this 66 year old lady with a long history of itchy ears, associated with ear discharge and a reduction in hearing. She has had a number of courses of antibiotics which offer only temporary relief.

Introductory question	**Answer**
What are the risk factors for developing otitis externa?	• Risk factors – skin conditions (eczema, psoriasis), instrumentation (cotton buds), trauma, water contact, occupation (dust eg. building site, musicians wearing ear plugs), secondary to middle ear disease (CSOM, perforated TM), foreign body, diabetes, malignancy.
Competency question(s)	**Answer**
On looking in the ear you notice a very narrow ear canal with infected debris. On	• Say at outset that the combination of OE in a 66 year old with granulations in ear canal make you somewhat suspicious and this merits careful attention. • **Complete the examination** to include neck palpation for lymphadenopathy and

microsuctioning you see some granulations in the outer half of the ear canal and you cannot see the ear drum. How would you proceed?	cranial nerve examination. • **Investigations:** ear swab, possible CT scan +/- MRI skull base depending on full clinical assessment. • **Treatment:** Initiate topical treatment for OE (Keep ears dry, consider antibiotic holiday if multiple recent courses, consider fungal infection and antifungal treatment. Regular follow up to clean ear until canal is patent and can see TM). However do not assume that this is the only problem there. - Consider malignant OE – admit, CT/MRI/WCC scan, iv antibiotics, hyperbaric oxygen, debridement, DM control - May need biopsy to exclude SCC
Advanced question(s)	**Answer**
Do biofilms play a role in chronic OE?	• **Biofilms:** dynamic structured network of microorganisms suspended within an extracellular matrix. Promotes antibiotic resistance and reduced antibiotic penetration due to elevation of minimum inhibitory concentrations to levels in excess of what can be delivered systemically. Topical antibiotic drops are delivered at higher concentrations locally but the polymeric external matrix of the biofilm reduces to some extent (but does not eliminate) the absorption of the antibiotic. Also the presence of beta-

	lactamase-producing strains of Pseudomonas aeruginosa increases in the biofilm state. Some biofilms also develop drug efflux pumps and this has been shown for ofloxacin. Super-resistant strains of bacteria have also been identified within the biofilm.
What is the role for surgery in OE?	Hence these factors predispose to the persistence of chronic OE. **Surgery in OE***:* For suction clearance under GA in children; for biopsy of suspicious granulations in ear canal to exclude SCC, or deeper lying polyps arising from middle ear or attic; consider bony and/or cartilaginous meatoplasty if canal very narrow (in some cases lining with a split skin graft may be necessary); in malignant OE may need surgical debridement if medical therapies ineffective and/or complications such as facial palsy exist.

4.16 VESTIBULAR SCHWANNOMA (ACOUSTIC NEUROMA)

SCENARIO **(followed by a clinical photograph)**	A 64 year old man presents with 6 month history of unilateral RIGHT sided high frequency tinnitus of increasing intensity. Recently, he developed severe hearing loss in his right ear. He is otherwise fit and well. On examination he complains of discomfort on insertion of the otoscope into his right ear, but the examination is normal.

Introductory question	Answer
Other than a Pure Tone Audiogram (PTA), what single investigation would you organise this patient?	• Magnetic Resonance Imaging of his Internal Acoustic Meatus (MRI CPA/ IAM). This is required to exclude a possible Cerebellopontine angle (CPA) lesion in any patient who presents with unilateral or asymmetric audiological symptoms, such as unilateral tinnitus.
Competency question(s)	**Answer**
This is a selected image from his MRI IAM series. What does it	• This is a coronal T1 weighted MRI scan with contrast through the level of the internal acoustic meati with gadolinium enhancement. On the right side is a

show? 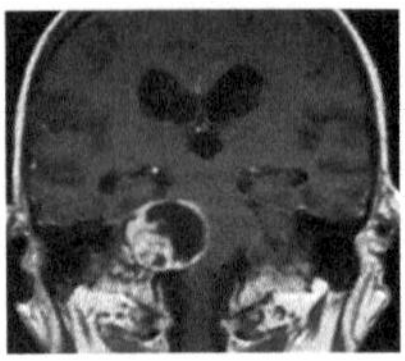	lesion with high and low signal in the cerebellar pontine angle. The lesion is compressing the pons. It is consistent with a vestibular schwannoma, which may have had a recent bleed into its substance, hence the sudden nature of the hearing loss.
What is a vestibular schwannoma and can you tell me a little more about this condition?	• It is a benign encapsulated tumour of the Schwann cells of the vestibular nerve. It accounts for 85% of all CPA lesions. They grow very slowly but are associated with a very rare malignant potential of less than 1%. Vestibular schwannnomas may be solid or cytic. • 95% are sporadic and unilateral and 5% are bilateral and associated with Neurofibromatosis Type 2, an autosomal dominant condition presenting with other intracranial and spinal lesions. • There are two histological subtypes; Antoni types A and B based on the uniformity of the cells. • They present classically with an asymmetric sensorineural hearing loss, unilateral tinnitus, vertigo and vestibulopathy, and facial weakness. Rarely they can present with central signs. • They can be treated by watchful waiting with serial scanning, stereotactic

	radiotherapy or surgery. Each case would usually be managed through a skull base multidisciplinary team.
Advanced question(s)	**Answer**
The patient complained of discomfort on otoscopy in the left ear. What could this represent?	• This is a positive Hitselberger's sign. This is an alteration of sensation to the posterior external auditory meatus or ear canal presenting with, discomfort, pain, numbness or paraesthesia of this area of skin. It is caused by a CPA lesion compressing, but not impinging on the facial nerve.
Aside from PTA and MRI, are you aware of any other investigating modalities that can be used for diagnosis (Historic examples accepted)?	• Speech audiogram showing rollover – a phenomenon where speech discrimination worsens with increasing sound intensity. • Stapedial reflex decay – an inability to maintain the stapedial reflex for 10 seconds in a sustained stimulus at 10dB HL. • Asymmetric caloric responses without any symptoms of vertigo. • Auditory Brainstem Response (ABR) – abnormal wave V latency between ears or abnormal interaural wave I-V and III-V latency difference.

4.17RAMSAY HUNT SYNDROME

SCENARIO **(with a clinical photograph)**	GP referral: Please could you kindly review this 69 year old man who noticed a sudden weakness of his face. 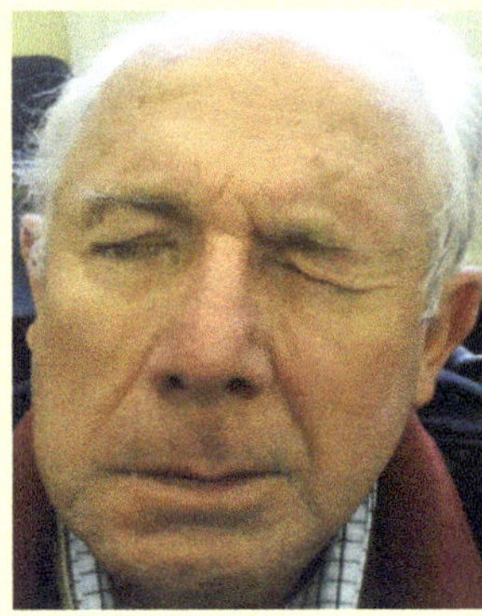

Introductory question	**Answer**
What are the key points to be covered in the assessment of a patient with a facial weakness?	• **History:** sudden or gradually progressive; any other associated neurological symptoms (speech impediment, arm/leg weakness); any associated vesicles; recent URTI or trauma or surgery; past history of facial weakness. • **Examination***:* Lower Motor Neurone (LMN) or Upper Motor Neurone (UMN) weakness (forehead sparing or not); brief

	neurological assessment; full cranial nerve examination; assessment of grade of facial weakness; examination of neck including parotid glands; examination of ears including tympanic membranes.
Competency question(s)	**Answer**
Assuming you have diagnosed a lower motor neurone facial weakness, what grading systems do you know? Describe the Sunderland system.	• **Grading**: • House-Brackmann (I - VI) is probably the most commonly used • Sunderland, (1st - 5th degree), Seddon (neuropraxia, axonotmesis, neurotmesis), Sunnybrook, Yanahigara, Sydney, Nottingham etc. • Sunderland System; - Conduction block only correlates with Sunderland (1st degree) and Seddon (neuropraxia) - Transection with intact endoneurium: Sunderland (2nd degree) and Seddon (axonotmesis) - Transection with intact perineurium: Sunderland (3rd degree) and Seddon (neurotmesis) - Above + disruption of perineurium: Sunderland (4th degree) and Seddon (neurotmesis) - Above + epineurium remains intact: Sunderland (5th degree) and Seddon (neurotmesis)

What investigations would you undertake? What is the evidence for the use of steroids and antivirals in the management of a LMN facial palsy?	• **Investigations:** Audiogram; CT temporal bones (either routinely or if abnormality on otoscopy); MRI neck/parotids if neck lump palpable; nerve conduction studies (not universally available). • **Evidence for treatments**: Scottish Bells Palsy study (NEJM, 2007) – early treatment with prednisolone is effective, whilst treatment with acyclovir is not. Likewise Cochrane review showed no benefit (2008). Various studies suggest that valciclovir may be more effective than acyclovir in combination with prednisolone.
Advanced question(s)	**Answer**
What surgical treatment is available for facial paralysis and when is it appropriate?	**Surgery** • If >90% axonal degeneration on nerve conduction studies. • Approach depends on which part of the facial nerve needs to be accessed and decompressed. Most likely site of surgical injury is 2nd genu but compressive effects of oedema most likely to be seen in labyrinthine and/or tympanic segments. Clinical assessment can guide to some extent the site of the injury – the presence of taste disturbance (chorda involvement), hyperacusis (stapedius involvement) and/or lacrimation (Greater

	Superficial Petrosal Nerve involvement) may determine whether a middle fossa approach is required for a predominant labyrinthine injury (although beware as hyperacusis is not thought to be a universally reliable marker of stapedius involvement as in some patients with hyperacusis, the contralateral stapedial reflex is still present). However Fisch (1985) reported good results with a combined middle fossa approach and mastoid decompression of the facial nerve in 11 out of 12 patients with Bells Palsy. **Facial reanimation** (static vs dynamic). • ***Static*** – gold weights, tarsorraphy, brow lifts, static slings. • ***Dynamic*** – temporalis transfer, XII-VII anastomosis.

4.18 MASTOIDECTOMY FISTULA

CLINICAL PHOTOGRAPH	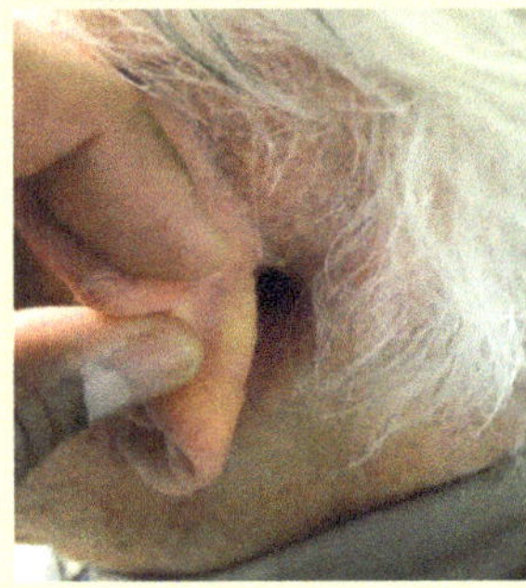

Introductory question	Answer
Describe what you see in the photograph	• This is a clinical photograph of a patient with a posterior auricular mastoid fistula. There is a clean, dry opening through the skin of the left post-auricular region. This is likely to communicate with the left mastoid antrum.

Competency question(s)	Answer
How is this situation likely to have occurred?	• This is a rare complication of mastoid surgery. • When a cortical Mastoidectomy has been performed and the skin wound closed, it is likely that there has been a wound dehiscence. This can be caused by haematoma, infection, inflammation or poor suturing technique. • It is more likely to occur in diabetic patients and smokers due to poor tissue healing. • Granulations growing through the skin wound can encourage a sinus to form.
What are the other complications of mastoid surgery?	Scar, Bleeding, Infection, Ear Discharge, Packs, Hearing Loss, Dead Ear, Alteration of Taste sensation, Facial paralysis (Temporary or permanent), Vertigo/dizziness, Tinnitus, Need for regular cleaning and water precaution, Recurrence.
Advanced question(s)	**Answer**
How would you manage this?	• Fistulas/Sinuses in this region are notoriously difficult to treat. In order to close this, a simple primary closure is unlikely to suffice. There is more likely to be a successful closure with a full

	thickness advancement or rotation flap from the adjacent occipital skin.

Also available:

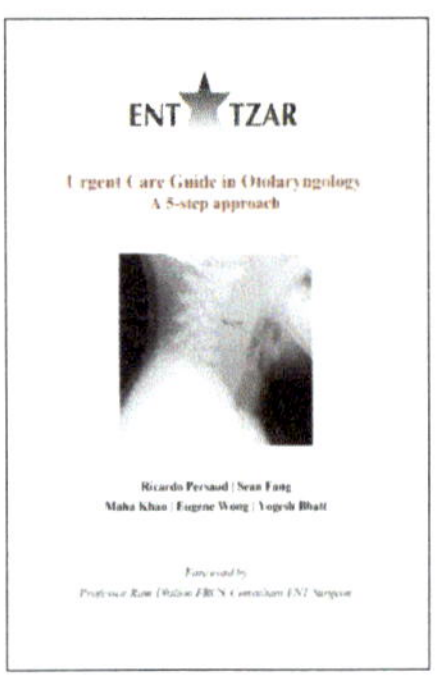

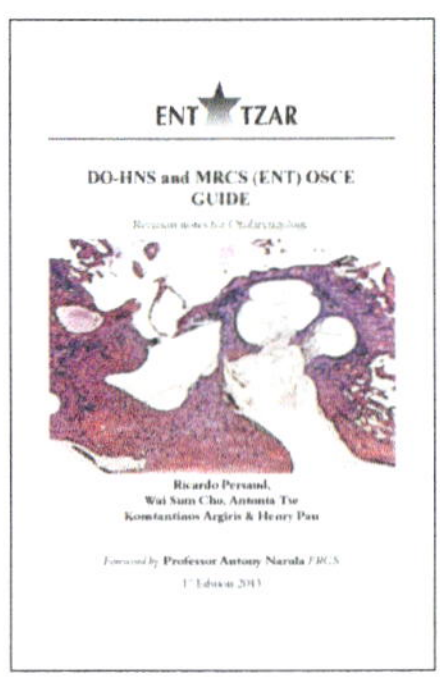

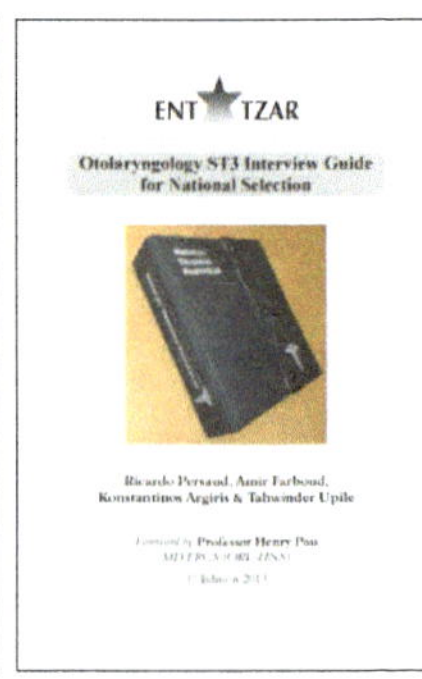

4.19 HIGH JUGULAR BULB

SCENARIO **(followed by a clinical photograph)**	A 38 year old man presents with a conductive hearing loss in his right ear. He was seen by the SHO in clinic and listed for a grommet insertion. Your registrar calls you to theatre during the procedure as he thinks the tympanic membrane looks abnormal. There is a 40dB conductive hearing loss and a type B tympanogram. 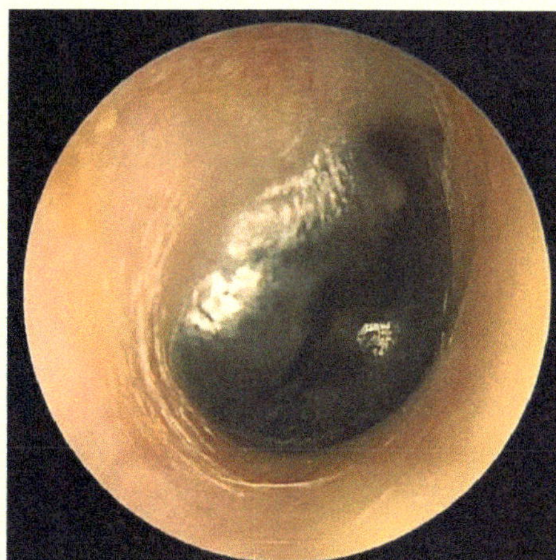

Introductory question	**Answer**
Describe this image?	• This is a clinical otoscopic photograph of a right tympanic membrane with the

	appearance of dark mass in the middle ear. This may represent a haemotympanum.
Competency question(s)	**Answer**
There is no history of trauma. What else could this be? What would your advice be?	• This appearance of blood behind the drum in the absence of trauma suggests a high jugular bulb or dehiscent jugular bulb. • Do not proceed with myringotomy and grommet insertion. This patient requires further investigation such as a contrast high resolution CT scan of the temporal bones. Treatment of the conductive hearing loss should initially be offered with a hearing aid.
Advanced question(s)	**Answer**
• What causes this appearance?	• A high-riding jugular bulb occurs when there is a congenital anomaly of the floor of the middle ear cleft, or a dehiscence in the floor. • The jugular bulb is the confluence of the lateral venous sinuses situated in the jugular fossa. It ultimately drains into the internal jugular vein passing through the jugular foramen. • At least half of cases are asymptomatic

	and are diagnosed only on careful otoscopy. • Symptomatic cases may present with conductive hearing loss, pulsatile tinnitus or rarely with facial palsy or vertigo secondary to erosion into the facial canal, vestibular aqueduct or posterior semicircular canal.
Had your registrar performed a myringotomy and called you for uncontrolled bleeding, what would you advise?	• Uncontrolled bleeding from a punctured jugular bulb is not uncommon as a presenting feature. The first manoeuvre would be to raise the head of the bed whilst applying direct pressure to the bleeding tympanic membrane. The affected ear should then be tightly packed with BIPP ribbon, adrenaline soaked ribbon gauze or gelfoam. The surgery should be abandoned. • If the bleeding is not controlled enlist the help of an interventional radiologist to attempt intravascular therapeutic embolisation.

4.20 GLOMUS TYMPANICUM

CLINICAL PHOTOGRAPH	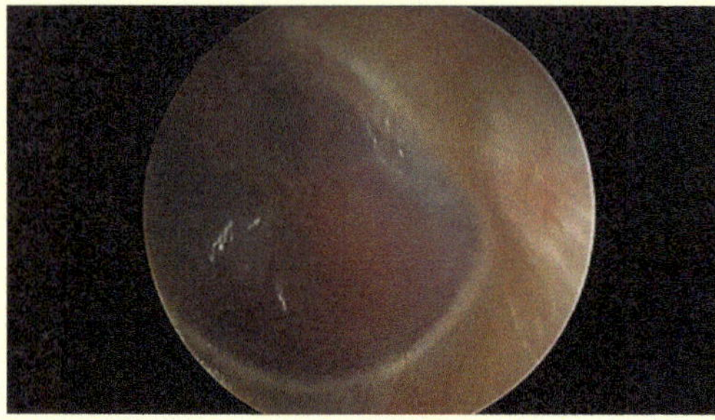

Introductory question	Answer
Describe what you see in the photograph.	• This is a clinical otoscopic photograph of a left tympanic membrane with a pink lesion occupying the lower middle ear space.
Competency question(s)	**Answer**
The patient presents with a pulsatile tinnitus. What is your diagnosis?	• This is likely to be a Glomus Tympanicum
What is a Glomus	• A Glomus tumour is a neuroendocrine neoplasm arising from neural crest cells of the parasympathetic nerves. They are also known as Paragangliomas or chemodectomas. They include Glomus

tumour?	Tympanicum, Glomus Jugulare, Glomus Vagale and Carotid Body Tumour. • They are highly vascular tumours supplied by the **ascending pharyngeal artery –** a branch of the external carotid artery. • Glomus tympanicum presents with pulsatile tinnitus and if extensive, may present with the effects of local erosion from the tumour. Other symptoms may include otalgia, hearing loss, vertigo and facial palsy.
What are the clinical signs found in Glomus tympanicum?	• In Glomus tympanicum, increased pressure on the tympanic membrane with pneumatic otoscopy will cause blanching of the tumour (Brown's sign). Pressure over the ipsilateral carotid artery will also cause blanching (Aquino's sign). • A CT scan can be used to assess size and bony erosion. An MRI scan is required to assess any intracranial extent of the lesion and classically shows a "salt and pepper" appearance on T2-weighted images secondary to the varying levels of blood flow. Angiograms may also be employed and can be both diagnostic and therapeutic if embolisation is used.
How would you investigate this condition?	• Urine and plasma catecholamines are measured to assess any concurrent pheochromocytomas.

	• 10% are multiple and are seen in Multiple Endocrine Neoplasia (MEN) type 2 syndrome.
Are you aware of any classification systems for paragangliomas?	• Yes, there is the Fisch and the Glasscock-Jackson systems. • Fisch - Type A – localised to middle ear - Type B – into mastoid (no bone erosion) - Type C – invades bone - Type D – intracranial extension • Glasscock-Jackson (Tympanicum) - Type 1 – limited to promontary - Type 2 – filling middle ear - Type 3 – extending into mastoid - Type 4 – extending into EAC or carotid • Glasscock-Jackson (Jugulare) - Type 1 – involves jugular bulb, middle ear or mastoid - Type 2 – extending under IAC with/without intracranial extension - Type 3 – extending into petrous apex with/without intracranial extension - Type 4 – into clivis, infratemporal fossa, intracranial.

Advanced question(s)	Answer
How would you treat this patient?	• Surgical excision can be achieved through a Tympanotomy using a laser for small lesions (Fisch Type A). Larger lesions may require transmastoid or infratemporal fossa approaches. • ENT surgeons operate on Fisch A-C with joint neuro-otologist for Fisch D. The intra-temporal fossa and translabyrithine approaches to the petrous apex do not require neuro-surgical input buth intracranial approaches do. • Pre-operative embolisation is often employed.
Why are glomus tumours so vascular?	• Because they secrete neuroendocrine pro-angiotic factors and enymes. They arise from angiotic neuroendocrine chemoreceptor cells which are associated with very vascular endothelium. • This is why pre-operative embolisation of the ascending pharyngeal artery may be appropriate in some cases.
Do they have a malignant potential?	• YES, in general paraganglomias have a 3-4 percent malignant potential. For temporal bone glomus, the figure is around 1 percent.

4.21 MENINGIOMA

Clinical photograph	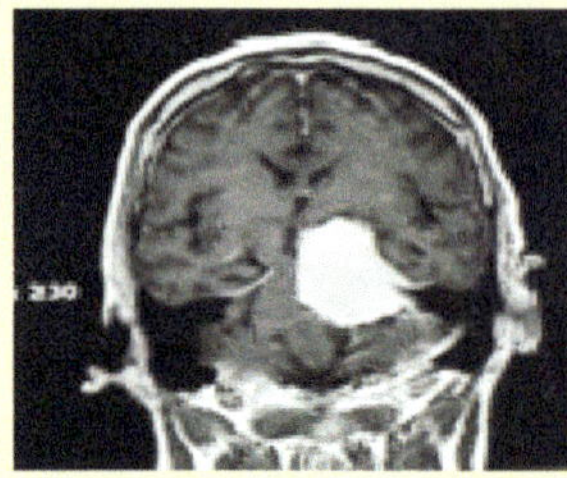

Introductory question	Answer
Describe the clinical image. What is your diagnosis	• This is a MRI of the brain and CP angle, coronal view. There is a huge broad-based mass in the left CP angle that is enhancing on T1 weighted image, post Gadolinium contrast. Dural tail sign is present, some element of compression of the cerebellar peduncle. • This is consistent with a left CP angle meningioma
Competency question(s)	**Answer**
What are the factors taken into consideration in managing these	**Patient factor** : Age, hearing status, fitness for surgery **Disease (tumour) factor :**

patients	Size, unilateral vs bilateral, compression on brainstem, operability **Surgeon factor** : Surgical teams available and preference (i.e. retrosig vs translab)
What are the surgical approaches for this tumour and the pro's and con's of each approach?	1. **Retrosigmoid**- preserves hearing, gives good exposure of CPA for large tumours, however cerebellar retraction gives constant headache post-operatively. 2. **Middle fossa** - preserves hearing, ideal for small intracanalicular tumours, however the temporal lobe retraction causes risks of fits especially in the elderly population 3. **Translabyrinthine** – facial nerve can be preserved, good exposure of the CPA however hearing destructive
Advanced question(s)	**Answer**
What are the categories of meningioma based on their sites of origin?	• Lateral • Mid-petrosal • IAM • Petroclival • Meckel's cave

4.22 BELL'S PALSY

SCENARIO **(followed by a clinical photograph)**	A GP has referred this 29 year old woman who noticed a sudden weakness of the face which shortly followed an upper respiratory tract infection.

Introductory question	Answer
What are the key points to be covered in the assessment of a patient with a facial weakness?	• **History:** sudden vs gradual, associated neurological symptoms (speech impediment, limb weakness), associated skin vesicles (?Ramsay Hunt), recent URTI or surgery, previous history of facial weakness • **Examination:** LMN vs UMN weakness (forehead sparing?), cranial nerve examination, assessment of grade of palsy, examination of the neck (?parotid mass), examination of the ear
Competency question(s)	**Answer**
What clinical grading systems of facial palsy do you know?	• Many grading systems described. • The House-Brackmann (I - VI) is probably the most commonly used

	• Other grading systems such as Sunderland (1st - 5th degree), Seddon, Sunnybrook, Yanahigara, Sydney, Nottingham etc.
Are there other methods of grading facial palsy more objectively?	• Yes, computer assisted systems e.g. the Glasgow Facial Palsy Scale (GFPS). This was developed by Mr. Brian O'Reilly as an objective method of assessing and presenting the house-brackmann and regional grades of facial palsy by production of a facogram.
What investigations would you undertake for a patient diagnosed with Bell's palsy?	• Audiogram • CT temporal bones • MRI neck • nerve conduction studies
Advanced question(s)	**Answer**
How would you manage a patient with Bell's palsy? 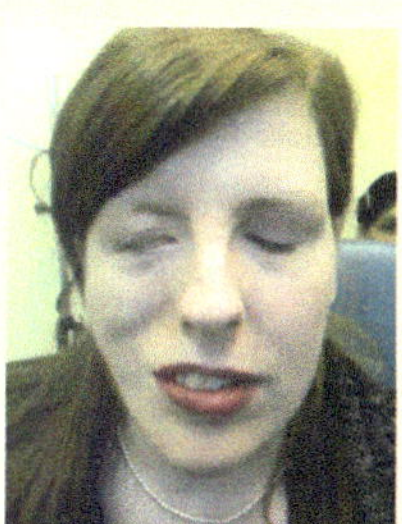	• Scottish Bell's Palsy Study (http://www.scottishbellspalsy.info/) *suggests that* early treatment with prednisolone significantly improves the chances of complete recovery at three and nine months. There was no evidence of a benefit from acyclovir given alone or of any additional benefit from acyclovir given in combination with prednisolone. • Cochrane review concluded that the available evidence from randomised

	controlled trials shows significant benefit from treating Bell's palsy with corticosteroids.
Would you consider nerve decompression in Bell's palsy?	• This is not conventional treatment and it would not be insensible to refer the patient to a neurotologist who has experience with this.A Cochrane review found that there was only very low quality evidence and that this was insufficient to decide whether an operation would be helpful or harmful for people with Bell's palsy. The authors suggest that there would unlikely to be further research into the role of surgery as Bell's palsy usually recovered without treatment.

4.23 CHRONIC OTITIS MEDIA ACTIVE MUCOSAL DISEASE

CLINICAL PHOTOGRAPH	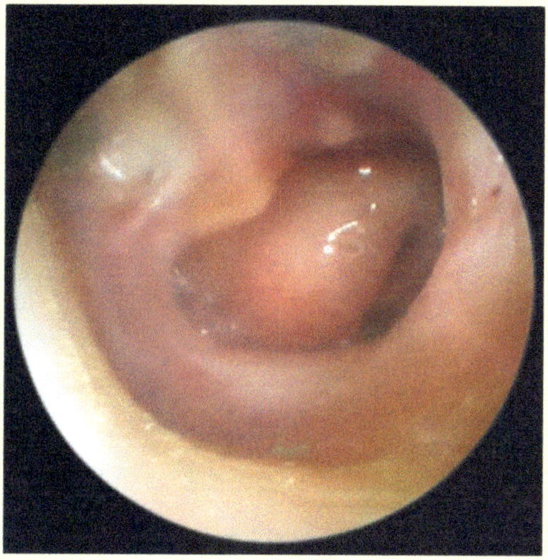

Introductory question	Answer
This patient is a 49 year old engineer with chronic discharge from ear nearly 12 months. Tell me what you see.	• Otoscopic view of the left ear with a large central wet perforation with possible erosion of the long process of the incus as the stapes head is visible. • The history and clinical findings are suggestive of chronic otitis media of the active mucosal type, although there may be an underlying cholesteatoma.

Competency question(s)	Answer
What is the pathogenesis of active mucosal chronic otitis media?	• Acute infection leads to inflammation of middle ear mucosa and oedema. Ulceration, granulations and polyp may follow because of breakdown of the epithelial reparative mechanisms. • The causative organism is usually pseudomonas (50-98% of cases); they use pili to attach to the necrotic/inflamed middle ear mucosa. Pseudomonas tends to release enzymes which inhibits effective immune response. Other organism implicated include s. aureus, proteus, klebsielly, diphteroids and fungi.
How would you treat this patient?	Investigations • Culture swab, CT if fails simple treatment, Audio. • Consider MRI if complications are suspicious. • 1). Topical antibiotic treatment/steroids • 2). Aural toilet • 3). Control of granulation tissue with silver nitrate cautery • 4). Water precautions • Associated nasal symptoms should be treated, eg with a nasal steroid and maybe a short course of anti-inflammatory antibiotics such as

	clarithromycin (500mg be for 7days).
Advanced question(s)	**Answer**
When would you perform surgery?	Indications for Surgery • Otorrhoea >6/52 despite appropriate antibiotics • Cholesteatoma • Coalescent mastoiditis

4.24a OTOACOUSTIC EMMISSIONS

CLINICAL GRAPH	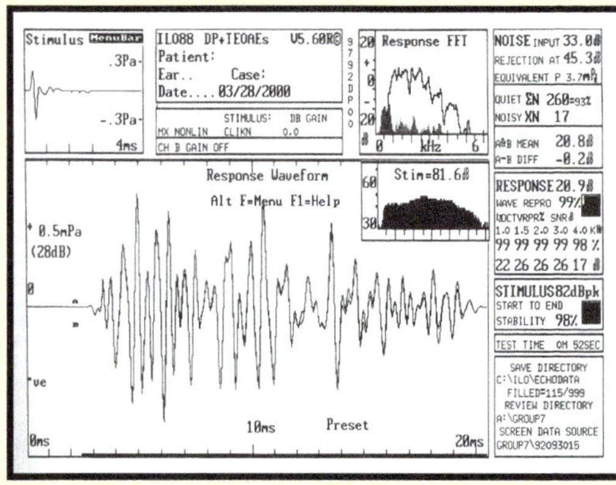

Introductory question	Answer
What is this graph?	• This is a graph of a transient evoked otoacoustic emmission
Competency question(s)	**Answer**
What does it show?	• I would like to highlight the stimulus, probe stability and the response in terms of the signal to noise ratio. • **S**timulus is good, ie, a broad band click (1.0 – 4.0kHz) that is clean, clear and has a positive and negative deflection, <1ms);

	intensity 78-86 dBpk SPL • **P**robe stability is good as it is >85% • **R**esponse: signal to noise ratio in dB across freq band is better than: Freq (KHz): 0.8 1.6 2.4 3.2 4.0 S:N (dB): 3 3 6 6 6 Clear responses present (i.e. Normal cochlear and middle ear function and Hearing thresholds better than 30 dB HL S:N in at least 3 of the 5 frequency bands needs to be equal to or greater than the levels shown above.
Advanced question(s)	**Answer**
What do you think about this graph? 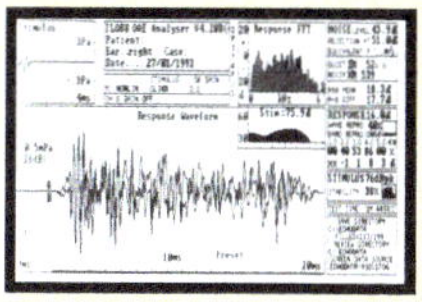	• Poor test conditions in terms of stimulus, probe stability and background noise. Therefore the it should be repeated. • Background noise can completely obliterate an OAE and interfere with signal to noise averaging. • Noise rejection • Probe fit should to stable, ie, tight to reduce background noise into the microphone • Baby state should be quiet and settled

4.24b OTOACOUSTIC EMMISSIONs

CLINICAL GRAPH

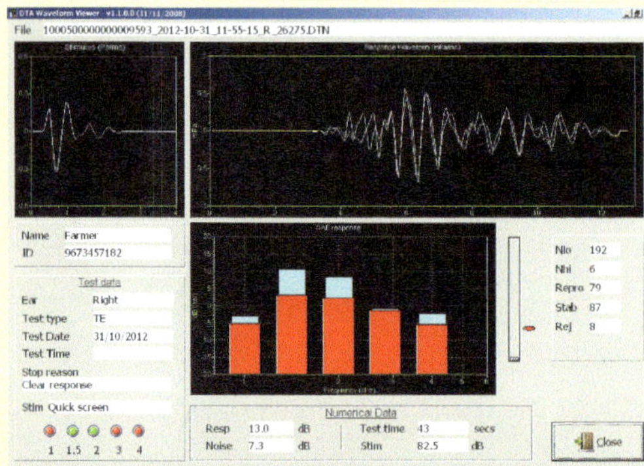

Introductory question	Answer
What is this graph?	• The new format of otoacoustic emmissions (OAEs) • It shows clear responses (Pass) because the stimulus is good, the probe is stable and at least 2 'signals' are above 6dB • In brief, 2 or more greens at the frequency 'traffic light' indicate a pass.
Competency question(s)	**Answer**
What are otoacoustic emmissions	• Small sounds generated by healthy outer hair cells either spontaneously or after a click stimulus (broad band 1-

	4khz)produced by tiny earphone for click stimulus. A tiny microphone detects OAEs • Patient should be still and quiet during recording • Impaired cochleae do not produce OAEs • High correlation between OAEs and normal audiometric thresholds (better than 30dBHL) • No correlations between size of OAEs and threshold level • Retrocochlear disorders not identified by OAEs • Important for Hearing screening, NOHL, Objective test for very young
Advanced question(s)	**Answer**
What do you understand about a click and a pure tone acoustic stimuli?	• A click stimulus is not frequency specific and consist of either a Narrow band (2-4kHz) or Broad or wide band (1-4kHz) • A pure tone stimulus is frequency specific; Tone burst and tone pips are the 2 types of pure tone acoustic stimuli; the former has an overall length >20ms whilst the latter has an overall length <20ms) **Additional info:** • Tone burst has a defined start (rise time), duration (plateau) and end (fall time); the

	plateau is longer than the rise/fall time. • Tone pips usually has a plateau which is the same or shorter than the rise/fall time.

4.25 UNIVERSAL NEONATAL HEARING SCREENING

CLINICAL GRAPH	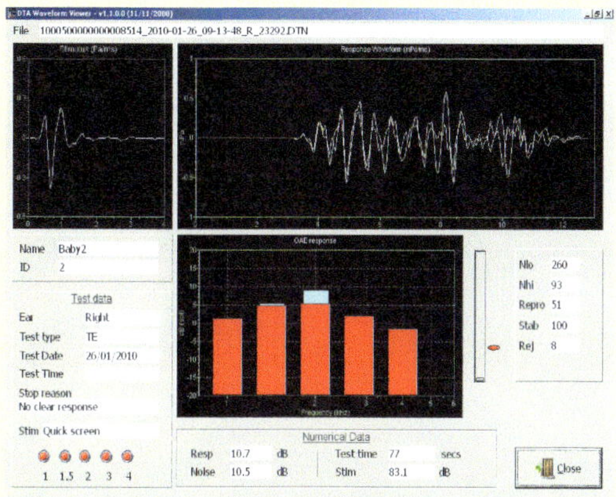

Introductory question	Answer
What do you think about the otoacoustic emission tracing?	• Despite a good stimuli and satisfactory probe stability there is no clear responses (Failed) (all reds at the frequency traffic light)
What is the aim of the Universal neonatal hearing screening?	• To identify PCHL>40dB in the better ear against a background of 1:1000 live birth in UK has permanent congenital hearing loss

	• 1st wave England 2000
Competency question(s)	**Answer**
Tell me about the screening tests. If the baby fails the screening process what happens next?	**Screening tests** • Normal well baby auto OAE and if the baby passes then screening is over. • If the screen OAE fails then it is repeat +/- with auto ABR (so the baby may end up having 3 tests: auto OAE, repeat auto OAE and auto ABR) • High risk babies: Auto OAE **AND** Auto ABR (High risk: eg nicu >48hrs, CF abn, infection, FH etc both OAE and ABR because of high risk of auditory neuropathy). • Referred via the Care pathways for DIAGNOSTIC assessment, Rehabilitation and Support.
Advanced question(s)	**Answer**
What is Auditory Neuropathy Spectrum disorder (**ANSD**)	Not a diagnosis but a name for a pattern of test results with • OAE/CM present • ABR absent or grossly abnormal at high levels And

	• Behavioural thresholds vary from normal to profound • Speech perception worse than predicted from PTA, especially in noisy environment Type 1-post synaptic ANSD • Nerve neuropathy • Dyssynchrony • aplasia Type 2-pre synaptic ANSD • Inner hair cells • Junction inner hair cell and auditory nerve

4.26 AUDITORY BRAINSTEM RESPONSE

CLINICAL PHOTOGRAPHS	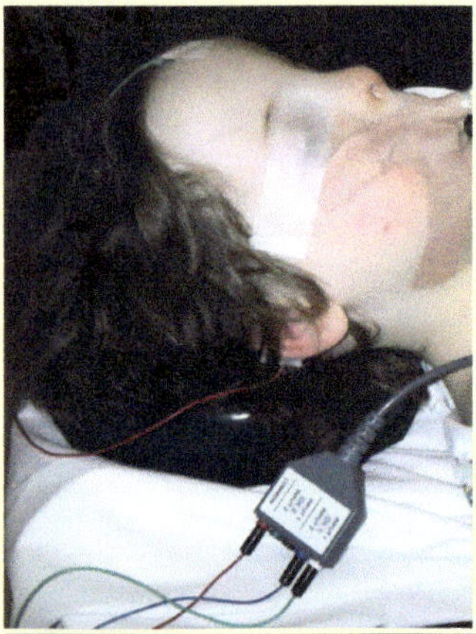 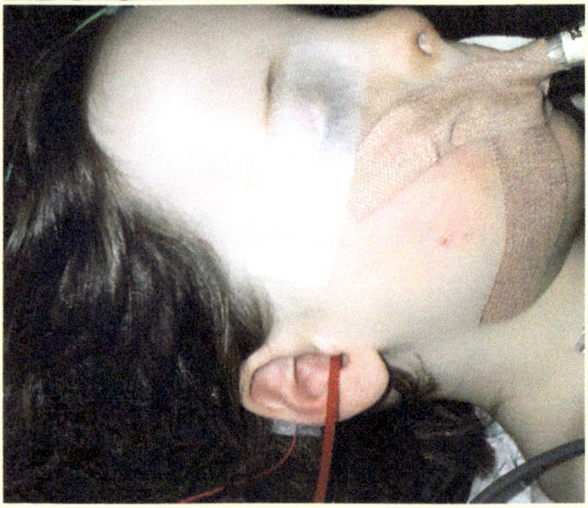

<table>
<tr><th>Introductory question</th><th>Answer</th></tr>
<tr><td>What investigation is being carried out on this child?</td><td>

- Diagnostic ABR (not automated ABR)

</td></tr>
<tr><th>Competency question(s)</th><th>Answer</th></tr>
<tr><td>What is ABR?

Tell me about this graph
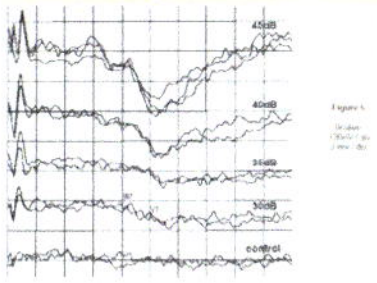
</td><td>

- Electrical response
- Generated by 8th nerve and brainstem
- Recorded via surface electrodes
- Typical morphology shown in printout with waves 1-5
- 1-10 m secs post stimulus
- Click stimuli are not good enough
- Tone pips @.5, 1,2,4 kHz used
- Small (50 nV) cf background noise
- Involves artefact rejection and Response averaging

- There is a clear response at 35dB
- There is also a clear response 5dB above (ie 40dB) but no clear response 5dB below (ie 30dB)
- The ABR threshold is therefore 35 dB

</td></tr>
</table>

Advanced question(s)	Answer
Explain what is a clear response?	Example of a clear response (*CR*), satisfying the 3 to 1 signal to noise criterion 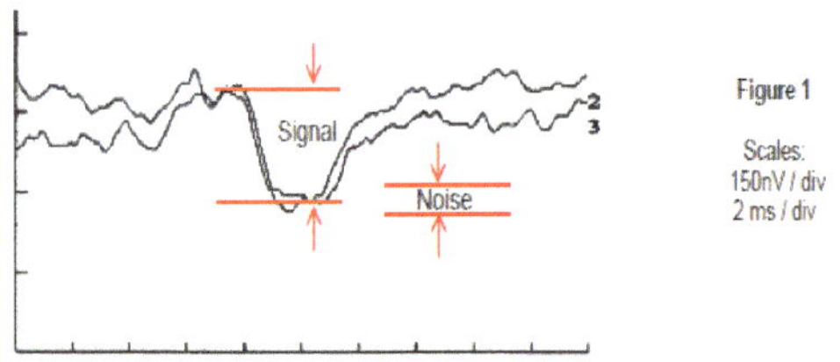
With regard to the age of the child what are the various threshold assessments available?	**Threshold assessment** • Less than equal to 6 months: **ABR** • Between 6 and 30 months: **V**isual **R**einforcement **A**udiometry • 30 months and above: conditioned sound field response (performance test), **P**ure **T**one **A**udiometry

4.27 PRESBYACUSSIS

CLINICAL AUDIOGRAM	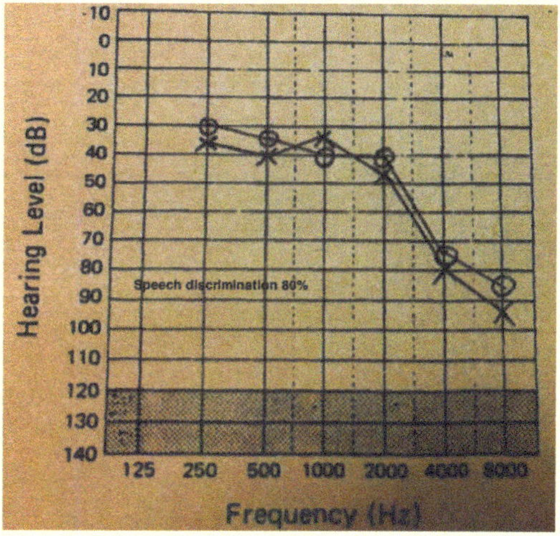

Introductory question	Answer
Describe this audiogram	• Bilateral sensorineural hearing loss • The pattern of hearing loss and the speech discrimination is consistent with neural presbyacusis.

Competency question(s)	Answer
What is	• Refers to the hearing loss experienced by

presbyacusis? What is the treatment?	elderly individuals. Important problem as elderly rely on hearing to counter deficits in sight & reaction time. In addition to decreased memory/concentration affects speech recognition (worse in noisy environments) 4 histopathological types • *Sensory* Epithelial atrophy with loss of HCs/supporting cells in organ of Corti (basal turn) possibly due to accumulation of lipofuscin pigment. Good speech discrimination • *Neural* Atrophy of nerve cells in cochlea and CNS pathways (?2100/35000 neurons lost/decade). Effects noted after 90% loss – i.e old age; Clinically disproportionate loss in speech recognition • *Metabolic* Atropy of stria. Flat HL with good speech recognition. 30-60 yrs • *Cochlear conductive* Thickening and stiffening of basilar membrane (good speech discrimination) Lip reading, air conduction HA, Assistive listening device

Advanced question(s)	Answer
What is recruitment?	• Recruitment is the abnormal perception of sound with small increase in intensity occurs in sensory presbyacusis (typically the patient says 'speak up doc I cannot hear you' and then when you raise your voice the patient says 'don't shout I am not deaf.'
How might the hearing aid audiologist deal with this problem?	• Clipping or compression
What would you do if the patient complains that hearing aids are inadequate?	• Assess for Cochlear implant

4.28 SUDDEN SENSORINEURAL HEARING LOSS

CLINICAL AUDIOGRAMS	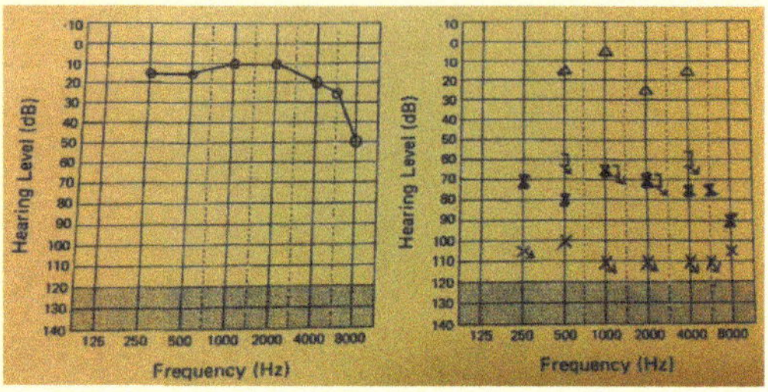

Introductory question	**Answer**
What is the diagnosis?	• Unilateral (left) sensorineural hearing loss • Normal hearing on the right, except 50 dB threshold dip at 8000Hz only
Competency question(s)	**Answer**
How would you defined sudden SNHL? How would you investigate and treat this patient?	• Sudden 30db HL in 3 contiguous frequencies for at least 3 days • FTA-Abs, ANA, RF, ESR, INR, aPTT, FBC – (infection), TFTs, Blood glucose, Lipid profile • MRI as 1-2% will have acoustic neuroma

	(3-12% acoustics present with SSNHL) • Audiometry If cause identified – treat otherwise • Carbogen (5% CO2) – vasodilator. • Increase blood flow (LMW dextrans, anticoagulants) – no supportive evidence • Steroids – systemic use supported by studies. Intratympanic for sever/profound • Others (antivirals, diuretics, hyperbaric oxygen) • Note spontaneous recovery in 47-63 percent of cases Negative prognostic Age <15 or >65; Eleveted ESR, Verigo or abnormal ENG; HL contralateral; Severe SSHL
Advanced question(s)	**Answer**
What is the pathogenesis of sudden SNHL?	4 theoretical pathways • *Viral infection* 17-33% patients recal preceding viral illness. Higher rates of seroconversion to HSV. Histopath evidence of viral induced damge to cochlea. • *Vascular compromise* Coclea = end organ. Function sensitive to b/supply. Time frame fits with vascular cause. Likely due to thrombosis/embolism/spasm/decresed

	blood flow. Risk factors similar to cardiac (hyperchol, low HDL,, high fibrinogen, smoking) • *Intracochlear membrane rupture* • *Immune mediated*

4.29 TINNITUS

CLINICAL PHOTOGRAPHS	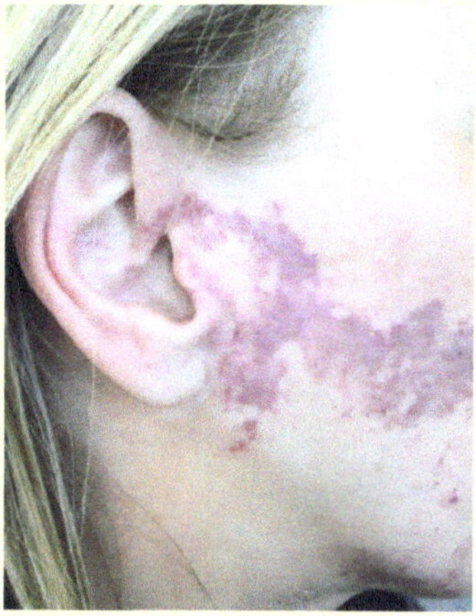 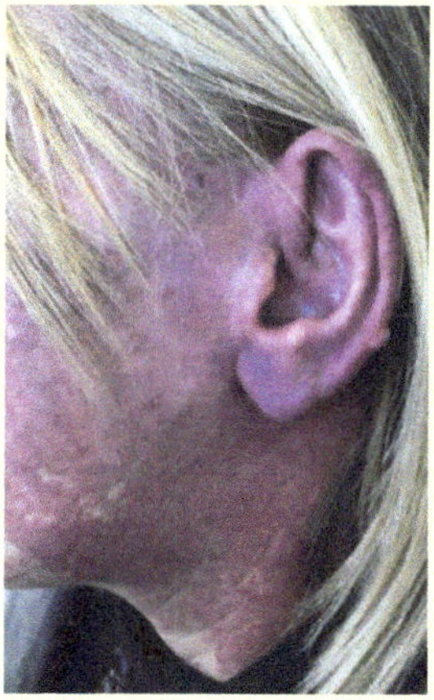

Introductory question	Answer
This patient complains of a pulsatile noise in her left ear. What is the most likely cause?	• These clinical photographs show a vascular malformation (rather than haemangiomas) affecting the face and therefore the cause for her tinnitus is likely to be vascular in origin, possibly arteriovenous malformation.
Competency question(s)	**Answer**
What is tinnitus?	• Various definitions exist such as the perception of noise in the absence of an external stimuli or an aberrant auditory phenomenon unrelated to an external auditory source or simply the sensation of sound arising within the head.
What investigations would you order for **pulsatile** tinnitus?	• Audiogram and tympanograms • FBC and TSH • Carotid dopplers • MRI/MRA head and neck • CT temporal bones
Is there any effective treatment for **subjective**	• Masking therapy (eg white noise maskers) appears to be effective • Tinnitus retraining therapy is also effective but no more than direct

tinnitus?	counseling. • There are other treatments but their effectiveness is controversial. However, there is evidence for favourable outcomes with benzodiazepines (eg clonazepam or alprazolam), antidepressants (eg amitriptyline, SSRI and tricyclic) as well as dexamethasone, but not for acupuncture, carbamazepine, Ginkgo Biloba or gabapentin.
Advanced question(s)	**Answer**
Have you heard of Tinnitology? Why do you think benzodiazepines may be effective in the treatment of subjective tinnitus?	• Yes, it started in 1987 as the study of how the perception of an aberrant auditory phenomenon can be translated into sensation and effect. • Benzodiazepines enhance GABA effects and may be effective because one proposed mechanism for tinnitus is the loss of GABAergic inhibitory neurons.

4.30 CLINICAL ANATOMY OF THE TEMPORAL BONE

CLINICAL PHOTOGRAPH	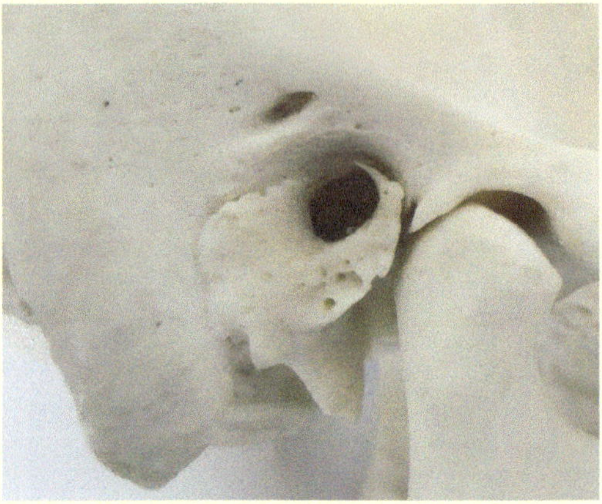

Introductory question	Answer
Describe the clinical anatomy of the lateral surface of the temporal bone shown here.	• **Lateral surface**: inferior temporal line, spine of Henle, root of zygoma, tympanic ring, tympanomastoid suture, tympanosquamous suture, TMJ, mandibular condyle and fossa, masoid bone
Competency question(s)	**Answer**
What is	• Macewen's triangle is formed by the

Macewen's triangle and its clinical importance?	inferior temporal line, posterior EAC canal wall and a tangential line joining the temporal line to post wall of EAC • It is a safe area to start drilling a cortical mastoidectomy as it is the lateral to the mastoid antrum and immediate behind the suprameatal spine of Henle – a reliable landmark. • In adults, the antrum is approximately 1.5 cm deep to Macewen triangle. • The antrum connects the middle ear cavity with mastoid and it is the first air cell of the temporal bone, formed by vacuolisation rather than pneumatisation, which produces the mastoid air cells. • Macewen area is the location of subperiosteal abscesses often seen in children; this is perhaps due to the porous-like cribiform plate of bone.
How might you prevent acoustic trauma whilst drilling the temporal bone?	• By not drilling near the ossicular chain, especially the short process of incus. • The short process of the incus and fossa incudus may be visualised early by utilizing the refractive index of water (remember temporal bone drilling should be sub-aquatic surgery).
Advanced question(s)	**Answer**

Where is Trautman's triangle and what is it significance?	• Trautman's triangle is the area bounded by the bony labyrinth (hard angle) anteriorly, the sigmoid sinus posteriorly and the posterior fossa dura (containing superior petrosal sinus) superiorly. • It is a potentially weak area through which an infection of temporal bone may spread to cerebellum. • A large sigmoid sinus may reduce the size of this triangle and also increase the angulation of the superior petrosal sinus. This potentially can impede the venous drainage and predispose to the development of endolymphatic hydrops (asymptomatic hydrops vs symptomatic hydrops). • The endolymphatic sac is located anterior to Trautman's triangle, medial and inferior to posterior semicircular canal (SCC).
How else might the endolymphatic sac be located during saccus decompression surgery?	• By using Donaldson's line, which is an imaginary line from Lat SCC bisecting (perpendicularly) the posterior SCC; it identifies the superior aspect of the endolymphatic sac.

Request from the Authors

Since there is always room for improvement, we would be very grateful for your constructive comments on this book. Please send your feedback via email to info@enttzar.co.uk or ricardopersaud@yahoo.co.uk . All comments will be taken into consideration whilst preparing the 2nd edition. You may also wish to consider writing a short review of this book on Amazon for the benefit of others.

Many thanks

RAPP | OJ | YMB | JAG | SCL | PC

www.enttzar.co.uk

9781784560874
ND - #0238 - 140926 - C382 - 197/132/21 - PB - 9781784560874 - Gloss Lamination